'This book is a burning manif[...] articulating shame and trauma. It is a testament to the feminist praxis of listening to each other's stories in collective solidarity as a refusal of erasure and a way to claim presence and power in the world.'

JESSICA ANDREWS

'A deeply affecting and eye-opening window into the world of shame, articulating exactly how you and others feel in a way that you may never have been able to say. Grace, style and empathy weave through this salient work.'

KIT CALESS

'A tender, intimate and generous meditation on the burdens of structural and personal shame on bodies and lives; and a radical call for the transformational power of speaking and listening.'

ELINOR CLEGHORN

'A potent depiction of abuse and transmitted shame – the type of shame inscribed on our bodies, clinging to our insides and concealed deep inside our core.'

NATALIYA DELEVA

'*My Body Keeps Your Secrets* will have forever shifted my perception of how shame works physically and psychically. Weaving her own personal experience with the testimony of others, Lucia Osborne-Crowley has written a singular work that I hope will inspire many more books like it. Imbued throughout with the author's potential for empathy, care and generosity, as well as her skill in both research and storytelling, this book is indeed a reclamation, through which we might reclaim ourselves from the shame of others.'

ALICE HATTRICK

'A deeply important book about the wide, deep ocean that is pain and trauma, about the reverberations through our lives individually and collectively, psychically and physically, that we are only just beginning to understand. How we can't separate our minds and our bodies; how it builds within us, even, maybe especially, if we try to disregard it.'

SOPHIE MACKINTOSH

'This book brilliantly interrogates our relationship to our bodies but also to those around us, inhabiting each daily, hourly, minute-by-minute contradiction that having a body, and so being alive, entails. A testament to the power of externalising our own stories so as to understand them through others' eyes, demonstrating how inextricably connected each of us ultimately is. Her writing is beautiful, unflinching and clear and, most importantly, it renders shame visible – a material thing that, having been sewn into the body, can also be cast off.'

OLIVIA SUDJIC

MY BODY KEEPS YOUR SECRETS

Dispatches on Shame and Reclamation

LUCIA OSBORNE-CROWLEY

THE

INDIGO

PRESS

THE INDIGO PRESS

50 Albemarle Street
London W1S 4BD
www.theindigopress.com

The Indigo Press Publishing Limited Reg. No. 10995574

Registered Office: Wellesley House, Duke of Wellington Avenue
Royal Arsenal, London SE18 6SS

COPYRIGHT © LUCIA OSBORNE-CROWLEY 2021

This edition first published in Great Britain in 2021 by The Indigo Press

A CIP catalogue record for this book is available from the British Library

ISBN: 978-1-911648-13-0
eBook ISBN: 978-1-911648-14-7

Design by Laura Thomas
Cover image © Arelix/iStock (after Matisse)
Typeset in Goudy Old Style by Tetragon, London
Printed and bound in Great Britain by TJ Books Ltd, Padstow

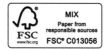

MIX
Paper from
responsible sources
FSC® C013056
FSC
www.fsc.org

CONTENTS

To everyone I interviewed for this book,
thank you for lifting me up with your bravery,
eloquence and grace. This is for you.

'What part of yourself did you have to destroy in order to survive?'

ALOK VAID-MENON, *Beyond the Gender Binary*

'What are the words you do not yet have? What do you need to say? What are the tyrannies you swallow day by day and attempt to make your own, until you will sicken and die of them, still in silence?'

AUDRE LORDE, *Your Silence Will Not Protect You*

'What is your aim in philosophy?'
'To show the fly the way out of the fly-bottle.'

LUDWIG WITTGENSTEIN, *The Philosophical Investigations*

REACTIONS IN THE AFTERMATH
a list in three parts

From Chanel Miller, *Know My Name*

I

0 hours to 24 hours after:

- · Numbness
- · Light-headedness
- · Unidentified fear
- · Shock

CHAPTER ONE

I read once that if you want to forgive someone for something – I mean really forgive – something has to die. That grief and loss and acceptance are necessary ingredients of truly letting go. I've been thinking about that a lot lately.

I've also been thinking a lot about philosopher Ludwig Wittgenstein's fly in the bottle. Wittgenstein said that systems of abuse are like putting a fly in a bottle. The fly can see out at the world because the glass is transparent. But the structure of the bottle is so vast and so consuming of the fly's small world that it cannot see the glass it is looking through; it thinks it is seeing the world as it really is.

And because the fly cannot see the structure imprisoning it, it is useless to say: You are in a bottle! The fly trusts that its perception of the world is real; to it there is no bottle.

All you can do is help the fly escape the bottle. Only from the outside, flying above it, will the fly be able to see what was imprisoning her.

The body is a very lonely place, especially when it is under threat. And some bodies are always under threat.

As I write this, the world is facing a crisis, the outbreak of the coronavirus.

The UK is in lockdown. Boris Johnson's government has closed all schools and cancelled GCSE and A level exams until further notice. The whole country has been ordered to work from home.

We are not allowed to go to friends' houses. All the bars, restaurants and cafes have been ordered to close. A few remain open for takeaways only, but anyone lining up must stand at least two metres away from other people.

This morning, I went for a walk on my own in the sun. I grew up in Australia, and I desperately need vitamin D to stay happy. It is a spring day in London, 23 March 2020. There is not a cloud in the sky, and there are daffodils everywhere.

As I walk through the clear air and look at the fresh flowers, I feel a strange combination of positivity and dread. This really feels like the end of days, but I am calm.

The streets are empty. The roads are empty. It is 9.02 a.m. Rush hour. But there are no cars on the road. The Tube station is closed, boarded up.

I walk past one corner shop that is open but there is a long queue outside, full of people standing alone and two metres away from one another. They all look slightly dazed. I wonder for a moment what I might think if someone dropped me here from another time.

I walk a few streets further to the Co-op. There is no line outside, but only because there is no food left on the shelves. All the big supermarkets have been ransacked and emptied out.

It happened slowly. The first thing to go was toilet paper – I still don't understand why, and that was weeks ago now. Then it was frozen ready meals. Then vegetables, dried pasta, tinned tomatoes. Coffee. Milk. Bread. Now the only thing left in my Co-op is Easter chocolate, which seems crass, the way it's all staring through the window at the street.

Last night, my friend and I went outside to see the International Space Station pass by. He has an app that shows him which planets and stars can be seen in the sky on any given night. The International Space Station can only be seen once or twice a year as it passes through a particular layer of the atmosphere. It sits thousands of miles above the earth in orbit. My friend looked on his app to see when it would be coming around next.

He gasped.

It's coming in twenty-four minutes, he said.

So, twenty-three minutes later, we are standing in the grass outside his flat, looking up at the sky. And then we see it. It looks just like a shooting star, only brighter. It moves through the sky quickly and then disappears after about ten seconds, into a different layer of the atmosphere, out of sight again. We both wonder out loud what the world will look like in 2021. Whether anything will ever be the same again. He asks if I think the people on the International Space Station know anything about coronavirus yet. Can they see us? Can they see that we've stopped going outside? Can they spot the cancelled sports and festivals and family lunches?

That's the best place in the world to be right now, he says. Quarantined in space.

Eighteen months earlier, I had moved to London from Australia. I was born in London, and had always wanted to find a way back here. I never would have guessed what would trigger the move.

When I was fifteen years old, I was violently raped by a grown man with a knife in an abandoned toilet in a Sydney fast-food restaurant. I thought I would die that night.

But I didn't die. I smashed a bottle over a toilet bowl to startle my attacker and I unlatched the door of the stall and I ran away. I ran and I ran and I ran. All I can remember is running. Down several flights of stairs, outside the restaurant, to where my friends were looking for me. We huddled together in a damp nook a few doors down and I slid down the concrete wall onto the floor.

I put myself in a taxi as fast as I could and I went home. I did not tell my friends what had happened, and they never asked. Because we were children, and we didn't know what else to do.

When I got home, I sneaked into my house via a side entrance to my bedroom with its en suite bathroom. I made sure my parents couldn't hear me.

I ran the shower hot and stood underneath it for a period of time that wore on endlessly. I was bleeding onto the floor of the shower and watching the blood drain away, hoping I could erase the memory of the rape with it. But it doesn't work like that.

At that time in my life, I was a very serious gymnast. I trained almost every day. I was in training for my second World Championships at the time of my rape. I made an excuse to skip training for a week so the bruises on my stomach and ribs could heal. I waited for the muscles in my pelvis to stop screaming and tearing when I walked. I waited for the joints in my wrists to stop aching. And then I went back to life as usual. I told no one. Not my parents. Not the police. Not my teachers. Not my friends. No one.

Eighteen months after my attack, I started having searing pains in my stomach and abdomen. They would come on unexpectedly but with such vigour, like a knife drawn through muscle. They became more frequent and I started collapsing from them. I started vomiting with the pain. I ended up in hospital again and again.

This triggered ten years of emergency admissions, tests and surgical procedures to try and figure out what had happened to me. The truth was there all along, but I couldn't see it. I couldn't bear it.

I was eventually diagnosed with endometriosis and Crohn's disease, both of which are – or could be – inflammatory diseases affecting the autoimmune system. Both often lead to chronic pain for the sufferer. Since 2009, I have been in pain just about every day. It never goes away for long.

When I was twenty-five, I had a breakdown. I am still not sure whether it was primarily physical or mental, but as I am discovering and rediscovering all the time, the distinction between the two is very slippery.

I became sicker than I had ever been. The pain was worse than ever and I developed intense tremors in my arms and legs. I was throwing up nearly every day, either from pain or the excessive doses of painkillers I was using to try and numb it. I lost seven kilos in two weeks. I desperately needed help.

So I decided to tell the truth about my rape for the first time. I told one of my therapists, and then one of my doctors. The house of cards began to fall, slowly at first and then very, very quickly.

Doctors told me it was very likely that my sexual assault was connected to my abdominal pain and my autoimmune illnesses. I started seeing trauma specialists who said the same thing.

I started doing research into the connection between violence and illness; violence and pain; violence and breakdown. What I found out was life-changing.

There followed months of appointment after appointment – with physical therapists, psychologists, psychotherapists, surgeons, masseuses, acupuncturists and sex therapists. The journalist in me decided to pretend that, during all these appointments, I was researching a story about someone else's sexual assault and recovery. I took fastidious notes. It was a way of keeping some emotional distance between myself and the heartbreak.

After months of this, I realized I had pages upon pages of notes, full of information I wish had been available to me earlier. I am incredibly lucky that I was able to go to all of these appointments – I had a job with enough income to cover them and lived in a place with a semi-functional public healthcare system. I am white and middle-class, both of which make it statistically more likely that I would be believed by doctors and given the appropriate treatment.

But the vast majority of people are not as lucky as I am, so I wanted to share the information I had access to as a result of those privileges. I started thinking about publishing the piece. I started showing it to trusted friends, and over the course of a few weeks, and with a lot of help, I decided to publish it in a literary magazine called *The Lifted Brow*.

Shortly after I published the piece, an editor in the UK commissioned me to turn it into a book. So I moved here, to London, on my own, to write that book. I thought my arriving here was the end of something hard, but it was the beginning of something harder. Writing that book – *I Choose Elena*, published in September 2019 – was by far the hardest part of my recovery.

I sat down each day trying to excavate my life, trying to pinpoint all the different ways this act of violence had impacted on me. But there was a problem: the book had to be about the rape and its aftermath, it had to have boundaries. It had to be confined to that. But the more I read and thought, the more I realized the rape was the tip of the iceberg. It was merely the most accessible – the most obvious – violation in a long story of intrusions, physical and emotional and psychological and familial and interpersonal, that make up one life in the body of a woman.

I moved to London to write the book because my publisher is based here, but also because I couldn't stand myself in Sydney. It was the only way I knew how to write those words down. It wasn't that I didn't have the support I needed; I did. I had it in spades. But something about my breakdown and the disclosure of my rape left me bitter and twisted and angry – three things I never wanted to be – and I felt I needed to get away to feel something new. I needed to put myself back together in a new way, in a new place.

I had very few friends in London. I had no doctors, no therapists. I was lost and alone.

I shut myself up in a small room and tried to make sense of things. As I was writing that first book, I read *The Lonely City* by Olivia Laing. A few friends who knew how isolated I felt had suggested it to me.

'You can be lonely anywhere, but there is a particular flavour to the loneliness that comes from living in a city, surrounded by millions of people,' Laing writes.

That's how I felt every day. I was shut up inside a small room, with barely any reason to go outside, ruminating on all the terrible things that had happened to me and the people I loved. Yet none of the people I loved were close by, so the tragedy felt deeper and deeper each day.

And then I read this:

'So much of the pain of loneliness is to do with concealment, with feeling compelled to hide vulnerability, to tuck ugliness away, to cover up scars as if they are literally repulsive. But why hide?'

I thought I had mastered the art of anti-concealment. I thought that by writing that book, I had vanquished my need to be invulnerable. I thought I had escaped loneliness by allowing myself to be seen.

But I hadn't. I was still ashamed. It was the everyday, insidious shame that hurt me most. The bodily shame that creeps into friendships and work and relationships and exercise. The kind that has both nothing and everything to do with my rape. The kind that I share with women and non-binary people all over the world who have, and have not, had experiences like mine. Their everyday shame also has nothing and everything to do with my rape, and with theirs. Shame and violation is a long-running war, and the everyday scars are the foot soldiers.

I spent twelve years thinking almost exclusively about my body. It was the only thing on my mind. As a semi-professional gymnast, I would be constantly appraising its power, its strength, what it needed from me, what it was asking for. Stretches, an ice bath, or maybe some extra press-ups to prime me for a competition.

Then I spent ten years not thinking about my body at all.

Because I had not told anyone about my rape, I had no way of understanding the acute dissociation I started experiencing in its aftermath. All of a sudden, my body felt so far away.

It was a crime scene, and I wanted to run from it and never look back. I started to ignore it, its sensations, its desires.

But the thing about living in a human body is that you cannot transcend it, no matter how hard you try. It is with you every day, every minute. You cannot leave it behind, you cannot change what it has seen and experienced. You just have to find a way to live with it. I know that now.

I have always been a perfectionist and a desperate overachiever. I thought I could challenge my mind to erase my assault and carry on as normal, in the same way I could challenge it to learn my English essays off by heart. But I was wrong.

As I was deciding whether to disclose my assault, I read a book by the psychiatrist Bessel van der Kolk called *The Body Keeps the Score*.

It is all about how the body remembers what the mind has suppressed. About how the body will carry scars of our experiences forever, no matter how badly we want to erase them.

That phrase just kept ringing in my ears for weeks. The body keeps the score. The body keeps the score. As soon as I read that phrase, I knew it was true.

One afternoon on a Wednesday in June, my therapist brings up the fact that I find an excuse to cancel our session every other week. My breath catches in my throat at this accusation.

I just mean, something always comes up, she says. Something always comes up that you are willing to put our session off for.

I stay silent for a moment, just a beat.

You pay for four sessions a month and only ever attend two, three at the most. You are paying good money in order to not see me on the days when you don't want to.

I don't respond.

And then she says, You are depriving yourself of care and, quite literally, depriving yourself of money that I know you don't have. Why is that?

I still have nothing to say.

I think there is a part of you that is still so afraid to be seen clearly by anyone, she says. Sustained contact is terrifying to you because it is the most intense form of exposure. The idea that I might catch you on a bad day really frightens you, because it means I will see that sometimes you are grumpy or underslept or resentful.

Or, she says after a pause, worst of all – when you are unhelpful. When you are angry. You are willing to be seen by me, but only when you feel able to curate yourself first. Only when you know you can say smart things and dutifully recount your week and encourage me when I make an observation that is accurate, only when you can be helpful and pliant and pleasant. This way, you are always in control. On the other days, you find an excuse to hide from me. You can't bear it.

She is absolutely right. I have worked so hard at expelling my own shame, but its grip is still suffocating. This woman, the person who knows more about me than anyone ever has, is still being presented a false version of me. I am still curating myself for her in order to hide the things I'm ashamed of.

But she has found me out.

Structural oppression lives and dies in the human body. Our tissues are its most elemental canvas. We have always known this, but we are still desperate to hang on to the idea that problems in the body are a matter of personal, not social, responsibility.

I grew up knowing in my bones that everything that went wrong in my body was my fault. When I was sexually abused as a child and I started getting chronic headaches each day that I knew I had to see my abuser, I believed there was something wrong with me, and not with him. When my body collapsed after months of ignoring pain from my rape as a teenager, I blamed myself. On the days when the pain of surgical procedures and side effects of medication get too much for me, I still blame myself, even though I know that so much of this pain was created by one man and his merciless, opportunistic crime.

The body is the beating heart of double-consciousness.

One body. That's all we get. One body that weathers every wretched storm.

When I started this book, I thought I was writing about personal stories. And I was, but I was also writing about something much bigger. What came out of my reporting is the story of countless systems of structural oppression, each of which enacts their worst consequences on the body we are forced to keep, the body we have to continue living in through every nightmare.

What came out was a story of structural discrimination, a scourge for which the blame is conveniently spread among the amorphous group, dispelled as responsibility spreads but for which the costs are felt in one body, felt sharply by each individual heart. The perpetrators are numbered in the billions – every person who upholds prejudiced structures of shame – but the most severe effects are carried alone.

When we see this clearly, we can ask ourselves: what does that do to a person? To a life? To each pound of flesh?

Almost all of the pain, suffering and illness recounted to me for this book is about keeping secrets. I first realized this when I started my own recovery from a rape I had never spoken of, childhood sexual abuse I had never admitted to, and the stress and toxicity that came from ten years of trying to outrun those basic biographical facts about myself. It occurred to me then that the thing that made me the sickest, the thing that made me suffer most, was the fact that I felt so compelled to hide what had been done to me. Because I believed it was my fault.

I wanted to test this theory, to see if it held true for other women and non-binary people too. People whose stories were more everyday than mine, more relatable. I spoke to almost one hundred women and non-binary people for this book, and in every instance my theory turned out to be right. Everyone I spoke to had either been dehumanized or had their personal dignity invaded at one point or another. They had all been made to feel afraid and then ashamed. They all felt they needed to stay quiet about the worst things that had happened to them.

The stories are all different, but their impact is the same. It's about the way we carry this impact with us. It's about the way we are taught to be ashamed of our own oppression. It's about gaslighting on the grandest scale. It's about feeling unable to speak the truth.

It is, in a single word, about shame.

Shame is the emotion that compels us to keep secrets. It comes from the outside, but it lives within. A very complicated demon.

Joseph Burgo, a clinical psychologist who has dedicated the best part of his career to researching shame, says in his book *Shame* that the emotion arises from a few key experiences. One is feeling exposed – that is, the fear of being seen. It's what my therapist was talking about that Wednesday a few weeks ago.

Another is unrequited attachment, love or affection. The shame of being rejected.

Another is failing to meet societal expectations – the burning shame of failing to fit the archetype you were born into.

Another is the feeling of exclusion based on some inherent rottenness inside of us. The feeling that we deserve bad things because we are fundamentally bad. That we deserve to be isolated, to be excluded.

It strikes me that those four categories can, between them, sum up every single story in this book.

All of those experiences lead to shame, and shame leads us to keep secrets, and secrets lead to suffering and illness and pain.

Here's another thing I learned. For most of human history, we have regarded emotions as a personal construct, things that appear in the privacy of our own minds in response to an external stimulus.

Something bad happens, and we instinctively feel sad or worried or anxious. By this logic, we punish ourselves and others for the emotional reactions we have. They belong to us, in some important way. We control them.

Women and non-binary people are again and again accused of illegitimately humouring emotional reactions that are deemed inappropriate to the circumstances. It is regarded as a personal failure if we overreact, if we feel too much.

But what if emotions are structural, too, and not personal? What if they are created by the world around us and also affected by shame?

Dr Lisa Feldman Barrett has recently published explosive research in her book *How Emotions Are Made* which, to my mind, confirms my theory. She has discovered that emotions are not the brain's private response to whatever external stimuli they are processing. In fact, the brain does not have enough time to take in the immediate stimuli. With so much going on – sounds, colours, bodily sensations – the brain chooses not to focus on analysing what is happening in that moment. Instead, it digests a few key elements of the situation – shouting, an increased heart rate – and immediately digs through all of its available memories about previous times when we reacted to similar experiences. It chooses the most relevant *set of experiences* and *constructs* and emotional responses based on those memories rather than concocting a bespoke response to each individual situation.

Here's what that means for my theory: rather than emotions being our individual response to any given situation, they are a mosaic of every similar experience we have ever had; a house of mirrors, each lurch of fear contains within it every fearful moment that came before it; every violation lives on inside the next, and the next, and the next.

So: we are not wholly responsible for the way we react to things. Our emotions are made up of a lifetime of experience of living in the body we were born with, and everything that comes with that. Once I cried on a second date – literally burst into tears without warning – because someone yelled at someone else at the bar and my brain interpreted it as violence. After that relationship ended, I couldn't stop thinking about that moment. How had I got it so wrong? How had I let him see how crazy I am?

But I am not crazy, and I no longer blame myself for that night. I interpreted that stimulus as violence because in my experience, that is what it has always been. Every woman in this book would have done the same. This is not my brain or my emotions malfunctioning, it is them responding appropriately to the body I have and the life I have lived inside it.

Once we accept that emotions are a constellation of experiences, we can see that they, too, are a product of structural oppression rather than individual weakness. Just like the illnesses and pain our bodies produce, we cannot be blamed for these vulnerabilities, because we did not choose them.

Because here's the thing. We all construct emotions out of memories. But some of us construct those emotions out of memories we cannot access and cannot talk about. We construct memories out of secrets. The worst things that happen to women, and those of marginalized genders, are kept hidden. That means our everyday lives, emotions and reactions are being dictated by a powerful force, a group of images and memories, that we do not understand – because we have never been allowed to talk about them.

That, I have discovered, can make us sick. It can make us anxious. It can make us sad. It can make us want to escape. It is a terrible, terrible tension.

In his book *Healing the Shame that Binds You*, psychologist John Bradshaw talks about chronic shame, or toxic shame. It's the kind of shame that comes from being told by society again and again that you are not good enough, that you are unworthy. It's the kind of shame transferred into our bones by a shameless act. It is the kind of shame passed down by traumatized mothers. The kind of shame handed to us by acts of violence and sexual entitlement. It is the kind of shame that gets under our skin through racist and sexist remarks in hallways and in knowing the next character assassination is always around the corner.

That kind of shame – the kind backed up by generations of human history and by tall men in oval offices and by school playgrounds and magazines – can become a way of life. It can become its own identity. If we are taught by the most authoritative sources that our lives are less valuable, then shame becomes a constant companion, and hiding who we really are becomes a way of life. It certainly did for me.

In this way, structural shame becomes personal. We act it out again and again and again, in everything we say and do and think. Because everything, at its root, can be explained by our conviction that we ought to keep hiding.

So we starve ourselves, and we out-busy ourselves, and we Instagram-filter ourselves, and we make ourselves sick, and we drink, and we escape, all to make sure no one actually sees us. All to protect ourselves from feeling exposed. From being found out.

To protect ourselves from the moment we let people see that the self we project is a lie, a curated image cobbled together by society's ideas about what a woman should be. That underneath all that is a real person, guilty of so many of the things we are taught to be ashamed of.

Guilty of having real, human skin and fat and cheeks and wrinkles and bones. Guilty of having needs – genuine, messy, human needs. Guilty of having feelings that ricochet. Guilty of being angry and sad and sometimes attached. Guilty of needing help. Guilty of having a body that takes up space in the world. Guilty of having been hurt in ways we may never recover from. Guilty of being raped. Guilty of being hurt by the people who were supposed to protect us.

Toxic shame is the voice that tells you that you are worthless. I know now that one of the effects of untreated trauma on the body and mind is to make us ashamed; to make us believe that we are, and always will be, people to whom terrible things happen – people who deserve to be hunted. This is put best in Meera Atkinson's *Traumata*: 'Shame is often transmitted, paradoxically, by shameless acts, acts in which one person's avoidance of shame demands another carry it.'

I haven't stopped thinking about that sentence since I read it. Shame is *transmitted*. That's exactly the right verb. Shame is passed from one human heart to another.

There is a moment in which one person decides to treat another with disrespect, decides to undermine that person's humanity and make them feel worthless. And in that moment, the predator hands his victim shame, and they are forced to carry it. Because that is the moment they start believing that there is something rotten in them; something that explains or justifies the predator's behaviour. We internalize the shame of a shameless act. It is the predator who has done the shameful thing, but they will never see it that way. Shame demands to be recognized, to be held. So because the predator refuses to hold it, we are forced to in his place. And it is from that moment onwards that we begin the project of trying to hide ourselves, so no one else can see the rottenness that the predator saw. Only the predator didn't *see* the rottenness, he created the rottenness. He *is* the rottenness.

Atkinson says of the man who abused her: 'I was ashamed for him yet it was not my shame.'

For me, that first transmission happened early in my life. I was nine when a man who was involved with my gymnastics club started sexually abusing me. His attention was my most precious thing. I adored him. He was truly godlike.

But he was quick to anger. If I did something wrong, or messed up one of my tricks, or tried to cut corners during training, he would scream at me. Really scream. He would yell and his eyes would water and his hands would flail about. I had no idea what it was about me that made him so angry.

But then when he was happy with me, it felt electric. The happiest I have ever felt. It was like magic. I wanted those moments so badly. I would have done anything to get more of them.

And when he was *really* happy with me, he would reward me with a private massage to soften my weary ankles and joints. And then those massages started to feel rotten. And then I was confused. I hated myself for making him angry, and I looked forward to the moments when I made him purr with pride. But then those moments started making me hate myself too.

I knew, I think, that the abuse was wrong. But I also knew that it was connected to his approval of me, and so I kept wanting it, even though I also didn't.

When you are treated like this as a child, it is very, very difficult for a child's brain to accept the fact that adults are not always good and caring. Especially if that adult happens to be one of your caregivers, which he essentially was to me. Because we cannot think of them as flawed, the only other cause for the bad behaviour must be us. We cannot say: This adult is bad. So instead we say: This adult is bad when they are around me, so I am bad. It's the only way we can make sense of it.

I became ashamed, for him, but it was not my shame. After that, those moments of transmission came again and again. When I was raped at fifteen. When men would rip my hair out during sex or try to strangle me or whisper horrific slurs in my ear. When boys at school teased me about tampons and sex and called me crazy. When boyfriends yelled at me and made me feel like I was evil. Again and again and again the transmission happens, until the state of shame becomes chronic.

Recently I told my therapist about a dream I had.

I am getting ready for training one morning before school. I pull on my leotard and bike shorts and wrap thick strapping tape around my ankles. Then I am crouching on the floor in a room I do not recognize. I am huddled over myself, my small arms wrapped around my knees and pulling them tightly into my body. I look down at myself in the dream. I am about twelve.

I am screaming: I don't want to go, I don't want to go, I don't want to go, don't make me go, please don't make me go.

An adult is standing over me, holding me, and saying: You don't have to go.

And the dream ends.

When I told my therapist this, I thought about all the times I cried in the middle of the night thinking about going to training the next day. About all the times I cried in the gym toilets before braving the session. I wanted so badly for it to end. I wanted so badly to find a way out.

But I never, never said to anyone what I said in that dream. I never, never told anyone I didn't want to go.

I just kept going, every day, again and again, swallowing my tears because I believed that I deserved the treatment I was getting from him.

I was the fly, and he was the bottle, and everything I knew to be true was refracted through his eyes.

I never left the gym, not until I injured myself so badly that my career ended. It was just after my rape. I hated it at the time, hated that my dreams had been crushed, hated that I had to leave. But when I think about it now, that injury seems cast in a different light. My mind wouldn't let me speak up, wouldn't let me say *he's hurting me*, wouldn't give me a way out. So my body did instead, and with that catastrophic injury, I was finally free.

Recently I told my therapist about another dream.

I am on a train, but one that looks like a hotel inside. I am sitting at a table, as an adult, drinking wine with this man, the man who abused me. Then, with no warning, we are off the train. Lying on the tracks together, as though we are about to get hit. As though these are our last moments.

He says: I'm sorry for what I did to you.

A long pause.

I say: Do you remember what happened on the train?

He says: Yes, I remember.

The dream made me think a lot about all the mixed-up memories I have of him. Some of them are clear, and I know that what happened was wrong. Some of them are less clear, and I still struggle to know what's real.

It makes me think of the writer Clare Best's words about her own sexual abuse at the hands of her father. 'I cannot reach some memories, or can only partially reach them, and that's both better and worse,' she writes. 'Better because I don't know exactly what happened, worse also because I don't know exactly what happened. Worse still because I know something toxic remains locked away.'

My therapist said something in that appointment that I keep coming back to.

You are always asking me what's real, she said. You are always looking for proof, something to show you what happened and what didn't happen.

I nodded.

But dreams are inventions of the subconscious. Every character in a dream is a part of ourselves. The man who abused you wasn't actually in that dream, wasn't in that conversation. It was just you. You talking to yourself.

Now say that dialogue again, she said, with that in mind. Say it out loud.

And I did.

Do you remember what happened on the train?

Yes, I remember.

In *Healing the Shame that Binds You*, Bradshaw says that when our lives get overtaken by chronic shame, we create a 'false self' to present to the world, one that we think is worthy.

Every story in this book is about how we learned the value of the false self, how we unlearned it, and the price we paid trying to attain it.

As the false self is formed, Bradshaw says, the authentic self goes into hiding. The false self is a masterpiece. Because the false self is an act of overcompensation for a part of us we believe to be damaged, he says, it is always more-than-human or less-than-human. 'It is crucial to see that the false self may be as polar opposite as a super-achieving perfectionist or an addict in an alley,' he writes.

Brené Brown says in her TED Talk that shame is an unbearable feeling, so we do whatever we can not to bear it. We escape it, we numb it, however we can. We become addicted to overachieving, to alcohol, to drugs, to sex, to toxic friendship, to starving ourselves, to hurting ourselves. These are all ways to numb shame. They are also, it seems to me, ways for the false self to punish us for being defective and carrying shame.

But Brown tells us something else that is very important about numbing shame: we cannot, no matter how hard we try, numb emotions selectively. If we allow ourselves to escape from shame, we also numb all the positive emotions we crave. We numb joy, love, safety, belonging, connection.

So the answer, I think, lies in finding a way to resist that escape. Brown says the best way to bear shame, without numbing it, is through empathy and connection. It's striking to me that she wrote this sentence in her audiobook *Men, Women and Worthiness*, long before the current iteration of the movement against sexual harassment was born: 'Want to know the two most powerful words when we are in struggle? *Me too.*'

It strikes me that the false self is also the key to understanding why I, and so many people in this book, struggle to know what is real and what is not; which parts of the world might be true and which are to be doubted.

Because we have always believed ourselves to be rotten and worthy of contempt, our own perceptions of the world are not to be trusted. All our lives we have been taught to lie in order to stay alive, and eventually we do not trust ourselves when we tell the truth.

My whole life has been either a paradox or a performance.

Gabor Maté, a physician and psychologist who works with addiction, eating disorders and other conditions brought on by shame, also has a groundbreaking theory.

Many long-term and chronic illnesses, including diabetes, dementia, autoimmune illnesses, arthritis and cancers can be a product of the impact of chronic and prolonged stress on the human body. In his book *The Body Says No*, he sets out a theory that almost all of those who develop these major illness have survived and suffered through physical or emotional trauma, and the stress carried in the body in the aftermath of this eventually causes disease.

This theory builds on Bessel van der Kolk's idea of the body keeping the score. Maté extends this theory to suggest that all different types of chronic physical and emotional stress can lead to serious illness. Perfectionism, overachieving, addiction, anxiety – all these traits can eventually make us sick. That is to say: trauma does not have to be life-threatening or even panic-inducing to live on in the body. It can be all the small traumas, pulled together in a constellation over a life, that can show up on the flesh.

The false self is hard work. The body is constantly in a state of fight or flight, afraid of being found out, afraid of being hurt again. Trying to pretend to be more or less than we are. Trying to prove something to someone, anyone. That causes the immune system and the nervous system to overreact and then exhaust themselves, after a lifetime of all that invisible labour.

Smoking cannot *cause* lung cancer. For that statement to be scientifically accurate, every smoker would eventually get lung cancer. This is not the case. Smoking combines with a number of other factors, including stress, to build up a mosaic that eventually starts to look like lung cancer. That's what Maté is saying. Of course chronic stress from trauma or from hiding doesn't cause serious illness. But it could be the tipping point between a person who gets sick and a person who doesn't. Did you know that, according to an article in Harvard Health Publishing by Laura Kiesel, 'Women and Pain: Disparities in Experience and Treatment', 70% of patients with long-term chronic pain conditions are women?

In some ways, Maté's theory can be interpreted as victim blaming: the way we choose to live determines whether we will become sick with cancer or brain disease or diabetes. This is not Maté's intention, nor is it how I read his research. But I'd like to add shame to this theory to further demonstrate why this research has nothing to do with how we choose to live.

All the behaviours Maté identifies – overwork, perfectionism, addiction, emotional repression – are all ways that we cope with chronic shame. They are all antidotes to feeling exposed, feeling excluded, feeling like a disappointment or feeling unrequited love. Those things are not personal failings, they are a symptom. They are just us coping with what has happened to our bodies in the best way – the only way – that we know how. They are ways that we keep the secrets of ourselves from the world. They are structural burdens; secrets we should never have to keep.

Here's what I learned in the years of research and reporting to confirm my theory: #MeToo allowed so many of the previously uninitiated to understand, to finally believe, that those obvious violations truly damage us. That sexual assault and harassment are not victimless crimes. That each act of invasion and violence is criminal and dangerous.

But here is what we have yet to metabolize: it is not just about the crime, but also about the cover-up. It is the years and years and years of hiding that come after the assault.

Sometimes what hurts us the most is the aftermath, the everyday challenge of living in a body that has been damaged and disrespected and shamed in some way.

Sometimes it is an illness that takes years to manifest. Sometimes it is breast cancer, decades after the rape. Sometimes it is PTSD, after too many suicide attempts, unacknowledged until the attempts are fully realized.

Sometimes it is an eating disorder from which we never quite recover. Sometimes it is anxiety that keeps us awake at night, and the physical breakdowns that come with lack of sleep. Sometimes it is alcohol dependence, which leads us to stumble into the road or wake up covered in vomit or that leads us to not wake up at all. Sometimes it is opioids. Sometimes it is depression. Sometimes it is chronic loneliness, enforced by our inability to be seen.

Sometimes it is the life we lost to a pregnancy we didn't feel able to terminate. Sometimes it is the life we lost to the child we wished we could have kept. Sometimes it is the life we lost to chronic pain that no one paid attention to.

Sometimes it is a death by a thousand paper cuts.

Here's what I want next from #MeToo. I want to move on from the men we call monsters and start talking about the greyer space. The smaller acts of shame transmission. The ones we cannot pinpoint because they do not have a beginning or an end: a jury's verdict, a healed bruise. They are just moments. They come and they go, and we think they don't hurt us, but they do.

I want to move on from the men we call monsters because I am tired of talking about them. I want to talk about *us*.

I want to talk about the moments after the shame transmission, the whole life that is lived afterwards, and how all the other shame transmissions cumulate until the false self is a necessary weapon. I want to connect the emotionally abusive boyfriend that we make excuses for to the boy who came before him who was too pushy at the party and to the Tuesday morning wolf-whistler who came after. I want us to understand that carrying other people's shame affects a whole life. I want us to keep watching the woman *after* the bad thing happens, after the secret has been locked away. I want us to see how it keeps affecting her even though she wishes it wouldn't. I want to connect the rape to the illness to the aggressive Hinge date to the screaming argument with a man you thought you were safe with.

Because once we do that, once we focus on the lives we live afterwards, we will be able to understand one very important thing that we are currently missing. It is not just the monsters who hurt us.

Once you look at the lives afterwards, you see that something can be only half-nasty, can be an accident, can be nothing more sinister than a man projecting what he has learned back out into the world, can be thoughtless. And it can still be ruinous. Those two things can be true at the same time.

I've always thought I had to prove something in order to make my suffering valid. Had to prove that the man in the toilets knew he had raped me, prove that he had planned it. That my gymnastics mentor knew I was too young for what we were doing. But I don't have to prove any of those things. None of us do. We just have to accept the damage that has been done to us by structural shame, the cumulative impact of every shame transmission, and allow ourselves space to let go of the false self, to take some time to rest. Then we can take it apart, piece by piece, once we inhabit our own lives, our real selves, again.

We now all know about Harvey Weinstein. We have imprisoned him both as a man and as a symbol. Sexual assault is now punishable in the world we live in. That is an incalculable victory. I am so indebted to the women who made that happen.

But here's what I want to do next. I want to tackle the harms that are harder to pin down. Our movement has campaigned on, and won on, the idea of personal accountability. I want to challenge it to do the same for systemic accountability. For all the days we wake up hating ourselves and do not know why. For the times when there is not a convenient figurehead to throw our spears at.

We are more reluctant to do this work because it is harder to find someone to blame. Everyone is responsible, so no one is. But I want this to be the next mountain we climb.

Just like our bodies and our minds, our illnesses and our emotions, oppression is not a personal act. It is a work of structural violence. Everybody is responsible. Everybody who perpetuates shame – and that is all of us – must now work to tame it. We must do that because then everybody who lives in shame will be able to ask: Which parts of myself have I buried in order to survive? Who would I be if I were not carrying around a false self?

Last night, the prime minister instructed everyone in the UK to stay indoors except for one period of exercise per day. The only shops that will remain open are pharmacies and supermarkets. Everything else must close. We can only venture outside with other members of our household.

So I am locked up alone in my apartment again, just like when I first arrived in London, but for very different reasons. With a pandemic just outside my windows, everyone has become acutely aware of their bodily functions. More so than ever. How fitting, then, to finish a book about bodies and shame when all around me our corporeal realities come crashing in.

For some of us – mostly for women and non-binary people – bodily awareness is commonplace. For others – mostly men – it is new. I watch the people around me adjust to becoming aware of their body's potential failings for the first time.

To have the body of a woman or a non-binary person is to be

constantly punishing and reimagining it. Like everything else, the structural impact of this pandemic will be gendered. Women and non-binary people will be less likely to be believed when they are sick or coughing, or when they complain of shortness of breath. They will be more likely to be infected with the virus because so many on the front lines of this war – healthcare workers, service workers, private carers – are women and non-binary people. As I mentioned above, women and non-binary people are also much more likely than men to suffer from chronic health conditions – one of the primary risk factors for deadly complications from Covid-19.

All because the frailty of the female form, the messy truth of it, is still perceived as something to be ashamed of, no matter where or how it makes itself known.

This is what the physicality of oppression looks like in 2020. This is how discrimination shows up on the body.

This is a story about all the things I am still hiding, and still hiding from. It is a story about all the ways that women and non-binary people are expected to keep the secrets of their bodies from everyone, even from themselves. About all the ways women and non-binary people are made to feel ashamed. About how, despite our best efforts, the body finds a way to express what the mind cannot.

Since I read van der Kolk's book, I have spent two years trying to help my body recover from my rape. But in that time, I have received hundreds of emails and notes from women and non-binary people around the world who are trying to reclaim their bodies, too.

This has made me want to test my theory that all the things we hold in our body, all the secrets we keep for other people, have a cumulative effect. That the body is a canvas. That everything shows up there eventually. That oppression has a physical dimension. That structural barriers take the body as their primary battleground.

That the body tells the secrets that we try to keep. The ones we keep from ourselves. The ones we keep on behalf of the people who have wronged us.

So to test my theory, I started interviewing women and non-binary people about how they feel about their bodies, to see if any versions of my own story came up in my research.

I put a few call-outs on Twitter and Instagram for interview subjects. All I said was that I wanted to speak to women and non-binary folk about their relationships with their bodies. I didn't go into anything more specific than that.

The stories rolled in. In total, I spoke to more than one hundred people for this book. I collected hundreds of stories about each person's life inside one body. I spoke to people from the UK, Ireland, Europe, Africa, Australia and Tibet. I spoke to people between the ages of thirteen and thirty-seven. I spoke to them for hours and days and months. The stories they wanted to tell me were about their bodies, but they were also about all the things we have to use our oppressed bodies to navigate: love and intimacy, motherhood, childhood, friendship, illness and pain. The story of the body is the story of everything. And for us, the story of everything is the story of shame.

A note on my reporting for this book: I have changed names and details when the subjects have asked me to, in order to protect their privacy and their wishes. When details have been changed, if the amended details present an image of someone familiar to you, I assure you this is a coincidence. I have also run each set of amended details by the subject to make sure they are comfortable with the new constellation.

The only selections I made between interview subjects for this book were to make sure I included every voice of colour, queer voice and disabled voice that I had access to and excluded some white, straight able-bodied voices in order to get the best possible balance of perspectives in this book. I did my very best to make sure in all of my call-outs and in all of my interviews that these people felt comfortable and necessary to this project. I did not reach out to anyone in these groups who had not volunteered to ask them to be included as a way to add more of these voices, because I do not believe it is right to pressure anyone into participating in a project like this. But what I can promise is that I prioritized giving space and attention to the voices from these groups who came to me.

Another thing I did not do as part of the reporting for this book was push subjects for any detail or information they did not offer voluntarily or were uncomfortable talking about. As a result, there will be gaps in these stories that you, as a reader, will naturally want me to fill. You will want to know more about the lives of my subjects, their families, their friends, their universes. Unfortunately, I cannot wholly satisfy this wish, although I fully understand it. I have made this decision because I know, from personal experience, how exposing it feels to offer your story to the public domain, and that feeling is allayed only by the knowledge that you did so from a place of agency and empowerment. If I pushed my subjects for details they didn't want to give, I would take away that agency and risk making this exposure harmful to them. So I ask you to consider the gift these people have given to us in being willing to speak about their shame, and take it as it is without needing more.

Each of these stories is true in its entirety and in its detail. I have not shielded you from the worst parts, although at points you may wish I had. I have done that for a few reasons. The first is that these subjects have trusted me deeply and wholeheartedly with their testimonies, and I believe it would be disrespectful to water them down. The second is that just as they trusted me, their audience, I in turn trust you, my audience, to hold these stories no matter how messy or uncomfortable they become. The third is that this project is, to me at least, meaningless if it does not accurately represent the truth of what I was told. The final reason is that shying away from the things we are afraid of is what caused the suffering depicted in this book in the first place.

My interview subjects told me details about their childhoods, their teenage years, their childbearing (or otherwise) years, and beyond. I have attempted in this book to reconstruct their stories into a chronological narrative that takes you on a journey through one life made up of a constellation of different stories and experiences, to show you the many ways shame can invade our lives and at how many different junctures it can appear.

Imagine what we could do with the time and energy if we decided to tell the truth about our bodies, if we were to reject the idea that a woman's body is designed as a canvas to construct an alternate truth and embrace the idea that it is designed to be a truth in itself?

In her book *Constellations*, the writer Sinéad Gleeson says:

> I am an accumulation of all of those sleepless nights and hospital days; of waiting for appointments and wishing I didn't have to keep them; of the raw keel of boredom and self-consciousness illness is. Without those experiences, I would not be a person who picks up those shards and attempts to reshape them on the page. If I had been spared the complicated bones, I would be someone else entirely. Another self, a different map.

Every woman and non-binary person carries complicated bones that they have been taught to believe are shameful. But they are not. The acts that make up these complicated bones – neglect, abuse, misogyny, objectification – are not these people's shame to carry. They are the beliefs and behaviour of shameless people who refuse to carry it themselves. So over centuries, things have become very confused. It is not women and non-binary people who should be ashamed. It is those who refuse to carry the shame. Our bones are not wretched in their complexity, but beautiful. They are testaments not to the worst things that have been done to us, but how we survived them.

This book is a testament to those complicated bones. I am glad I am not a different map.

As I realize that the body shows us, ultimately, what we cannot see, or what we refuse to see, what we cannot bear to see, something else occurs to me. It seems to me that to live in the body of a woman or non-binary person is to never be quite sure about what is real and what isn't.

In her memoir about abuse at the hands of her high school teacher, *Being Lolita*, Alisson Wood writes about the moment her teacher whispered to her: *Secrets are safe.* That is what all abusers and people who hold power would have us believe. It is what I believed for all of my life. As Wood said later in an interview about her book in *Bomb* magazine, 'Secrets felt familiar, and so I believed the teacher when he said they would keep me safe.'

But it's not true. Secrets are deadly.

I am sitting in my old psychotherapist's office while I am on tour in Australia with my first book. It is the first time I have visited Sydney since the day I left to write the book, the day I escaped. It has been eighteen months since I saw my Sydney therapist, the one who started all of this, the one who saved my life.

I am here because, the night before, I had a panic attack about my book. About my weight, about my face, and about how punishing myself for not looking good enough was a way of punishing myself for writing a book that was not good enough.

Kamal takes care of me so well. He talks me through what happened and he gives me something to help me sleep and to keep the fear at bay.

I should be better by now, I tell him.

What do you mean?

Why am I still doing this?

He smiles at me.

Two weeks later, I am back in Sydney on the last leg of the book tour and I see him again. In those two weeks, he has read my book, a copy I gave him in that first reunion session.

I think your book will save lives, he tells me. I think it will be an important work for a long time.

He is crying. So am I.

But there is so much you haven't said, he says after a pause. There is so much more than what is within these very boundaried pages, he says as he holds up the book.

I know, I say.

There is all the nuance, he says. The stuff you still don't understand.

I know.

That's what you need to try and tackle in your next book.

I know.

It will be much, much harder than this one.

I know.

Adrienne Rich writes in her book *On Lies, Secrets, and Silence*:

Women have been driven mad, 'gaslighted' for centuries by the refutation of our experience and our instincts in a culture which validates only male experience. The truth of our bodies and our minds has been mystified to us. We therefore have a primary obligation to each other: not to undermine each other's sense of reality for the sake of expediency; not to gaslight each other… When a woman tells the truth she is creating the possibility for more truth around her.

CHAPTER TWO

I t is January 2019. I wake up sleepy and overwhelmed and heavy and I wonder how long I have hated myself. I am afraid to see my own, untouched face in the mirror that morning – the one with imperfect skin and tired eyes and day-old mascara and unbrushed teeth and pyjamas that are wholly unflattering but necessary to defend myself against the London winter. I brush my teeth without looking in the mirror. This is a studious exercise. It is harder than it sounds. It is a skill I have been working on for ten years. It is an achievement that no one will ever recognize; a craft I have always known I needed to learn but one I also must never speak about.

The hatred I feel about myself on this particular morning is the nagging kind. The kind that demands attention. It is the whimper of an unattended pet, hungry and wanting and desperate and uncompromising. What am I to do with it? How can I distract myself from it, or, better yet, numb myself against it?

It is 7 a.m. and I have to ready myself for the day. At some point I will need to go outside, to be visible, to be seen, to occupy the world. How am I to do that?

I pull on Spanx that feel as though they might squeeze me to death. I have recently been baking – a hobby I am told is healthy and mindful, and one I find incredibly calming. But it also means I have put on weight, means that my thighs look different, pale and under-attended. So I must hide them.

I dress all in black. I have always done this. When I was twelve, I read in a teen magazine that it was 'slimming'. I have never looked back. I often dream of being a girl who walks the streets in sunflower dresses.

I apply my make-up as though I am Vincent van Gogh. I apply the parts that are supposed to look organic, to look as though your natural skin shines like the moon when caught at the right angle. Then I move on to the parts that are designed to look fake, to look enhanced and hyperreal; the ones that prove to the world that I have made an effort. These elements are in deep conflict with one another, but both are essential. I have always known that. I study my face in the mirror to ensure I have struck an appropriate balance between the two. This part is crucial, a high-stakes endeavour, yet at the same time I find it is easy. I am playing the first game I learned.

I take a photo of myself with an Instagram filter that makes me look less pale, one that hides the scratchy effect of a long winter on the skin. I snap picture after picture after picture, wondering whether people will notice the extra weight on my face. I try every angle I can think of until I find one that makes my face look thin. I adjust my skin tone a bit more – this is the black clothes of the make-up world; it sheds weight like magic. I experiment with facial expressions – do I want to appear earnest, as though I believe I am beautiful, or impatient, or as if this whole endeavour is a vacuous joke? Do I smile? Do I roll my eyes to express my internal conflict about the painful act of self-curation I have just undertaken as the very first activity of my day, as I do every day? Do I look at the camera or away from it? Am I the kind of person who looks at the camera? What kind of person am I? What am I doing?

I post the photo. It is now 8.30 a.m. and I will be late for work. I sit on the bus as it trundles down Stroud Green Road and I wonder what my boss will think about my lateness. But then it happens – the first push notification of the day. Someone has liked my Instagram post. Then another someone, then another. Each one is a shooting star, finite but endlessly captivating. Each one is a heartbeat. It is my heartbeat; it is the only thing telling me I am alive, or perhaps the only thing telling me I deserve to be. I am twenty-seven.

On a mild September evening, I am sitting in a cafe in Finchley with my editor. We are meeting for the first time and we find we are instantly animated, talking about bodies, and shame, and secrets, and pain; talking about all the things we are not supposed to talk about.

I tell her how badly I want to write about teenage girls, how I admire them so much. Girls who have to live in the world as young adults in 2019 are facing a tumultuous uphill battle. They are so brave. They are taking on the fight against their own oppression in ways I never did at that age, and the world was so much easier for me. There was no Instagram, no Snapchat, no revenge porn, no unsolicited dick pics. Just Internet Explorer and MSN Messenger. The most dangerous the internet ever got for me was the boy in my class who said, 'Wanna cyber?' one day right before I closed his chat window.

But girls today, it's a whole different story, I say to my editor. Instagram is full of tips for throwing up your food. I tell her how I used to trawl the internet for advice – I was a terrible bulimic for months and months before I got the hang of it – and all my searching back in 2011 turned up next to nothing. It's so dangerous now, I say. And it's so time-consuming. Did you know, I ask her, that girls spend an average of forty-seven minutes a day taking selfies?

In response, she asks me if I've heard about the face editing apps. I nod. She says she knows some women her age, in their fifties, who use face editing apps before posting photos of themselves on Facebook and Instagram. We note that young people do this too. People my age who won't post a selfie until they have spent hours editing it, making their eyes brighter, their freckles dustier, their face more contoured.

Secretly, I am one of those young people. I edit my photos every day. When I'm not happy, I send them to my sister's partner – a graphic designer who is brilliant at using editing apps – and get him to edit them for me. I quite literally post professionally edited photos on my Instagram story feed and pretend they are candid and of-the-moment.

I think about the uphill battle I am describing among these teenage girls I pretend to have authorial distance from. I wonder if I am in the same battle. I wonder if I am losing. It's time to go and meet Emma for our interview.

.   .   .

Emma is fourteen when I meet her. She is moving schools. It's the middle of the school year. When term breaks up for Christmas, she won't be coming back.

The sun was shining despite the frost when she woke up on her first day of her second to last week. She thought about the girls who tormented her, the ones she wouldn't have to see again. She thought about the way the other girls talked about her, the way everyone knew her as the loud one with all the opinions. She thought about how she wouldn't have to think about that any more.

But then she thought about the boarding school she would arrive at a month later. She thought about how no one would know her, about how perhaps that was worse than what she had faced already. She thought about how the girls would watch her walk in on her first day, about how they would study her fourteen-year-old face and body. What would they think? The empty space after that question mark had been haunting her all week. She had been at her school since she was four years old. Never moved. Never been the new girl. Better the devil you know.

As she walked down towards her bus stop, she caught her reflection in the mirror. Her hair was curly and wild. She liked it. But her body felt and looked heavy, burdened. She thought that she was still too chubby, too round. Too sloppy. She doesn't need to be perfect, she thinks. She's not asking to be a supermodel. She just wants a break from this feeling, like she is always taking up too much space. When she explains this to people, they rarely understand. All the adults' faces harden or become vacant, they are uncomfortable.

But you are so thin, they say in hushed tones.

Don't talk like that, Emma.

Stop it.

How could you think that?

Stop it.

Don't be silly.

But she isn't being silly. She is being honest. She wakes up every single day and wishes to be different. To be smaller. To be lighter on her feet. Why will no one listen? She isn't asking anyone for anything. She isn't asking them to sign a solemn declaration confirming that they agree that yes, she is chubby for her age and yes, she should lose weight. She is just asking for the space to talk about it. Why is that so hard for grown-ups to understand? What are they afraid of? Why are they so afraid?

All Emma wants to do is lose a stone by the time she starts at her new school. Technically, her BMI tells her she is overweight. She just wants to get down to seven stone. Then her BMI will be average, and she will be happy. That's all she wants. To be average. To be happy.

When Emma says this to me in 2020, I shudder because I know that BMI calculations are inaccurate and misleading and cause so many girls to hate themselves. And I shudder because I am twenty-seven and I still check mine almost every day, knowing I will be happy when it comes up with the answer UNDERWEIGHT and then the words DO NOT USE THIS TOOL IF YOU ARE BEING TREATED FOR AN EATING DISORDER. Some habits die hard.

In class that day, Emma thought about how she would lose weight. She had one month of holidays. She was due to start at the new school at the end of January. That's plenty of time, she thought. She would exercise every day and she would eat healthily and she would limit the time she spends on screens. She would eat raw carrot for breakfast instead of toast. She would go for long walks every day while listening to her music.

When the bell rang at the end of science class, she walked quickly towards her group of friends. They were fairly new, this group, and they were not so bad. The year before, she had a falling-out with the girls she used to be friends with. She was not sure if she would ever get over it, if she was honest. It was torture. Girls can be so cruel.

But the new group was different. They were much more like her. Edgier. They were artists too. They were not vain or superficial and they were not obsessed with Instagram. She might even miss them when she left.

She saw them standing in the usual place, between the drinking fountains and the towering archway. One of them was slouching against the wall, telling a story. The rest were listening intently. Before she reached them, one of the girls from her English class tapped her on the shoulder. She was tall, and slim, and beautiful.

Here you go, the girl said, offering a bundle of pages held together by a paper clip.

Thanks, Emma said back. Because she was leaving, Emma had mentally checked out of this school. She hadn't been paying attention in class. So she'd been getting the other girls to give her their notes in exchange for drawing lessons.

She has been teaching herself to draw all year. She is quite good at it, she thinks. It all started with her obsession with anime. She started drawing all the characters, and she wanted to get better, so she started studying the art of drawing anime in her free time. Then she moved on to abstract portraits, then onto realism. Then she moved back to abstract. You have to learn the technique before you can throw it out the window, she remembers an art teacher telling her once. Only once you have mastered the complexity can you make things simple.

She tells me about how she plans to lose the weight in that time: eat less, exercise more. This, too, is simple, she says.

It doesn't sound all that simple to me. She is a child. I stare into her eyes and I wonder how this could have happened, how the world could have taught her that she is so unworthy of it already.

She tells me it all comes from a period in her life a year or two earlier, when she was very depressed.

Everything stopped making sense to me, she says. My mental health just crumpled.

She is so articulate, so clever, that sometimes, when we talk, I wonder if someone is playing a trick on me. Whether someone has somehow put a grown-up's voice into this small girl's body to confuse me, to derail my book project.

She tells me that when she got really, really sad, she started overeating.

I just ate and ate and ate, she says. I couldn't stop. I just sat all day eating and snacking, sitting in front of a screen, never getting up.

She tells me that she gained weight quickly, without noticing at first. By the time she noticed, she says, the problem was out of control.

I had put on so much weight that I couldn't stand to look at myself, she says.

After a pause: I still can't. But I'm going to be healthy about it this time. I'm just going to cut out screens and do more exercise and eat healthier. I could be eating a banana right now, but I'm not. She motions with the carrot she has been munching on while we've been talking.

Because I am a journalist, I have been trained to understand how to make people feel comfortable in a conversation. I have been taught how to show an interview subject that I am listening, that I am with her. I have been trained in the art of asking questions. Of asking the right follow-up questions at the right moments. Leaving the right pauses in the right places. Nodding. 'Mmm'-ing. I have been trained in the art of making people feel seen. Or perhaps I have this the wrong way around. Perhaps I became a journalist because I had already been trained in these things. Perhaps I am a journalist because I am a woman.

But interviewing Emma causes me to question every instinct. As I automatically go to nod along with her, to make encouraging sounds, I keep thinking: How can I do that when a fourteen-year-old girl is sitting in front of me talking about needing to lose a stone in a month? How can I, in good conscience, nod along as if this isn't extremely alarming to me? How can I hide from her that I, too, fall into the category of grown-ups she is talking to me about, the ones who baulk at her need to be smaller, who tell her to stop, who are afraid of her illness.

What are they so afraid of? she keeps saying to me.

What am I so afraid of, I think. Am I ashamed? Is it my shame or hers? Do I say something? Do I give myself away? Or am I just here to observe, to render this problem into something concrete without intervening in this moment. Is that all journalism can do? Is it enough?

.   .   .

When I was Emma's age, I was separated from the boys in my school's basketball team and I was not sure why. I asked a teacher and he told me that boys were better at basketball than girls, but I didn't believe him. He said my body was different to theirs, which I understood was partly true, but I didn't understand the significance of this difference. I was an athlete. I competed in national championships for gymnastics and frequently won. Why couldn't I play sport with the boys?

It's not appropriate, he said.

I didn't really understand this either, but I gave up and went back to playing with the girls. My body was nothing to me at this time. It was neither comfortable nor uncomfortable. It just *was*. It helped me with my gymnastics career and it burned when the skin rubbed off my palms from too much time on the uneven bars and it throbbed when I twisted my ankle but other than that I didn't think about it very much at all.

It was incidental, which is to say it was fine the way it was. It wasn't something I thought about, which is to say I did not feel the need to change it. It was a fact of my life, as banal as all the other facts of my life at that time.

At home, there was no one to talk to about bodies. It was simply not something that ever came up in our house. I was aware that my private parts were private, but no one ever told me this. I was never told how my body works, what it is made up of, or what – or who – to protect it from. It was never spoken about outside of conversations about gymnastics. We discussed sprained ankles and sore muscles and missed landings, but that's it.

I was happy with this arrangement. I felt like it was right that I didn't know. There was something very fundamental in me telling myself that it would be shameful to know, shameful to think about, shameful to acknowledge, the truth of my body. Somehow I knew it was more proper of me to pretend it was not there. And that's what I did.

I only started to see my body, I mean really see it, through the eyes of others. At age eleven, the boys used to pass around notes in class with the names of all the girls in the room and a column to rate their looks and personality out of ten. Once all the girls had been assessed and graded, the notes were passed to us so we could see how we'd done.

This was a cruel exercise, of course. But I didn't mind it because I poured all my energy into being the nicest of the nice girls, polite to a fault, saccharine sweet, soft and malleable and easy.

I always got ten out of ten for personality, and that's all I cared about. When I say that's all I cared about, I am not trying to pretend I was being subversive. I was twelve. It was genuinely the only thing I thought to be important.

But when the following school year started they added a new column for 'body'. I know this sounds ridiculous, the clinical nature of it all, the clean break between childhood and adolescence, but that is genuinely how it happened. Something changed that summer. It had been a long, dry season in Sydney, my school friends and I had started going to the beach together, and the boys had started commenting on our bikini choices.

I went to a mixed school with a much larger proportion of boys than girls, so we were around boys a lot. There was no time or space for us to discuss these issues without them watching. That summer they started watching.

As soon as they started asking questions of us, we started asking questions of ourselves. One of the boys taught me the word 'cellulite', which I had never heard before. We started repeating the comments they made to us in our locker rooms on sports days and at sleepovers and in the line at the school canteen. It seems strange to say this now, but it is not even a slight exaggeration to say that the very first words I learned to describe my body were the ones formed in the mouths of boys who were criticizing it.

I don't know if it's something about growing up in a city full of beaches, but the bikini conversations felt like the beginning of it all for me. I suddenly became aware of a whole new world that I had never considered. Something I was being judged on that I didn't know how to improve. Something my kindness and pliability could not shift.

.   .   .

Back in Emma's living room, I ask her what she means by 'this time'. She has just said, I don't want to be unhealthy in the way I lose weight, this time. She tells me about the last time she tried to get slimmer, when she was depressed and barely left the house. She would sit for hours and hours on Instagram, looking at what she calls ED content. Eating disorder content. She would only follow the people the ED community call 'skinny legends'. Girls who track their illness by posting photos of their own disappearing acts, posting long captions with tricks for how to throw up food soundlessly, how to pretend to chew and eat in public, how to stop yourself from finishing any meal by forcing yourself to eat it in front of a mirror. She tells me how addictive it was, knowing there is an endless amount of uncensored content on there for her to mine. Every day there were new posts, new tips. She knew it was unhealthy, she tells me now. She knew it was making her sicker. But it also made her feel like she was part of a community. It made her feel less alone.

So I'm avoiding that part of Instagram this time, she says.

I wonder how it could be that, at thirteen, she had already gone into this tunnel and come out the other side. I shake my head, and then wonder if this symbol of disbelief might give me away.

.   .   .

As I leave Emma's house and walk towards the Tube, I am still thinking about the head-shaking. And then I start thinking about why I am so alarmed.

Because she's so young, I keep saying to myself. She is a child.

And I think about myself at thirteen, and I realize I was deep into my own eating disorder by then. To people around me, I probably looked just like Emma did to me. I looked like a child, because I was one. But not to me. Not in my head. In my head, I had already fought and won a thousand battles with my body. Worrying about all the ways it needed to be different, concocting plans, failing at them, punishing myself, starting again. Rinse. Repeat.

When I get home, I write down the ED hashtags Emma told me about so I can find the corners of Instagram she took refuge in. I scroll for hours through posts more horrifying than I could have imagined, and again I wonder whether it is right or wrong, helpful or harmful, to reproduce these images with my words. The hashtags are full of pictures of girls posing in front of mirrors, looking close to death, spindly and small and breakable. Pictures of wrists and ankles and clavicles that are nothing but skin and bone. Posts sharing weight loss tips and purging tips and places to hide uneaten food.

I hadn't heard about ED content before I met Emma. I knew there were parts of Instagram and Tumblr that allow anorexic girls to connect with each other, but I had always naively thought the purpose of this was shared healing. What Emma was telling me was something very different. It was about shared joy. About shared accomplishments.

About egging each other on. I don't know what to make of this. It swirls around and around in my head between my own carefully rationed meals.

I decided to write this book because I wanted to test my thesis about lying with the body, about how this sits at the heart of suffering for others as it has for me. But here's what I didn't expect: for those who came after me, those with more and more and more media with which to promote the lie, it is worse.

In her essay about recovering from an eating disorder, 'The Quickening', the author Leslie Jamison writes:

> In the years since those days of restriction, I have found that usually when I try to articulate this to people – *I felt like I wasn't supposed to take up so much space* – they understand it absolutely or not at all. And if a person understands it absolutely, she is probably a woman.

I think about that imperative, the need to take up less space. It is connected to the need to be superhuman, to be not-quite-real, to be curated and preserved in our best form. Staying small, starving ourselves, is one way of doing this, but really every story in this book is about taking up less space in the world.

Self-harm and our desire to hide our suffering, inflict it on ourselves before it escapes into the world. Beauty standards and Instagram filters and our desire to be uniform. Hiding our abortions and our miscarriages and our traumas and our crushed dreams. Overachieving and embracing perfectionism so that we never need help, a constant commitment to hiding in plain sight. It all comes down to the same thing. Wishing to be invisible, knowing that we will ultimately be punished for allowing ourselves to be otherwise.

Listening to Emma makes me think so much about the first time I realized, at least consciously, that I needed to change myself in order to fit in. The first time that urge became a compulsion.

When the boys introduced the 'body' column into the notes, my success plummeted. I would still get glowing reviews for my personality and average ones for my looks, but my body really let me down. I was getting twos and threes and fours. As a Type A overachiever, I was absolutely shocked. How could that be? As with anything I did back then, I started paying attention to the criticisms because I needed to get my grades up. I was so eager for approval.

Although I had spent most of my childhood not thinking too much about my body except in its athletic capacity, once I did turn my mind to the question I decided that my body was pretty good. Great, even. I loved it. I looked at it in the mirror before going to the beach and I thought about all the nice things the boys would say about me in their heads. This was not arrogance, I don't think, or bravado. It was just a quiet acknowledgement that my body would be well-received. I was wrong.

When the twos and threes and fours started rolling in, I was horrified. The boys told me I was too muscly, that my six-pack from ten years of gymnastics training was disgusting, that I was flat-chested and looked like a boy. They started to point out the muscles in my arms when I lifted my school backpack and flung it over my shoulders. They looked inside my school shirt and saw that I was wearing a sports bra while the other girls were wearing underwires, because I hadn't developed yet and I had nothing to put into those cups of theirs. I was so ashamed.

I started obsessing over my body in the mirror every day after school, before school, during school and wondering how I could fill it out. I eventually bought bras and stuffed them, and I started avoiding swimming in front of my friends so they wouldn't uncover the deceit. I read online that eating chicken helps women put on weight, especially in their waist and hips, so I started eating chicken for every meal. I did this for a year. Fifteen years on, I am still an A cup, but I'm okay with it now. In those years, though, I spent so many hours trying to figure out how to expand myself. A few years later I would develop anorexia and become obsessed with restriction, with making myself disappear.

In those later years, I felt sick when I thought about the chicken project, that I had wanted there to be more of me.

CHAPTER THREE

Every time I think about my conversation with Emma, I can't help but think about how early we are taught to pretend to be different than we are. It is so deeply ingrained in childhood that by early adolescence we are already working on lying with our bodies. On creating a canvas out of ourselves rather than a human body that lives and breathes and moves and fails and lets us down as often as it doesn't.

The body we are born with is never allowed to just *be*. It must be curated and changed until it feels like a mask, like something we can disappear behind, like armour. A false self. This seems to be so fundamental to the experience of being a woman or living outside of the gender binary.

Emma saw that her body was starting to reflect her sadness, so she had to change it. She saw something that, to her, seemed to be imperfect or flawed and which was connected to her fractious state of mind. By trying to lose weight again, she could go back to feeling in control of herself and her life. She could morph into the person she wanted to be, rather than morphing her wanting to reflect the person she actually was. We didn't speak about why this was – whether she had asked for help and been denied it, or whether she didn't feel able to speak up at all.

This seems to me to be, at its core, about shame. It's about this idea that the truth of our bodies must be hidden, that we must not be found out. That we must always be hiding, be projecting a version of ourselves that is controlled and curated and contained. We have been taught that that is the way to break free of the shame we are made to feel. We have been taught that we will stop hating ourselves, stop being ashamed, if we just change ourselves. But it doesn't work like that. Shame is nebulous, shape-shifting, it has no finish line.

I have spent my whole life trying to numb the things I am ashamed of by changing the way my body moves through the world. I have lied about my illness to try and quash the shame I feel about being a failure. I have lied about my 'natural thinness' in order to numb the shame I felt after my rape, thinking that staying stick-thin would offset the deep self-loathing I had been left with. That if I changed myself, I could change the facts of my life. That I could change the terrible things that had happened that had made me feel as though I wasn't real, as though I didn't deserve a complicated, human existence.

In *On Lies, Secrets, and Silence*, Adrienne Rich talks about the way women are taught to lie with their bodies in order to protect themselves from the world. They are taught that this works, but it doesn't. The truth bubbles over eventually, and the consequences of the lie can be lifelong.

.   .   .

I am thinking about Adrienne Rich's comment when I meet Rowan, who is nineteen and only four years out of a long stint in an inpatient psychiatric hospital for people with severe eating disorders. One of the first things she says to me is: *I am as recovered as I will ever be.* Even now, she believes this. The cost of the lie will never go away, not really. The damage we do to ourselves for the temporary numbing of shame can be permanent.

Rowan was fourteen when she started starving herself. She was in year nine at her high school on the outskirts of London. Whenever she tried to stop the deprivation she was putting her body through, she couldn't. Towards the end of that year, she started engaging in escalating acts of self-harm. She was admitted to an inpatient ward for teenagers with severe eating disorders when she was fifteen years old.

It was the only way to be physically safe from myself, she tells me when we meet in 2020. She is now nineteen.

When she first arrived on the ward, Rowan was told she would stay for six weeks. She was placed in a small room with a small window. She was forced to put on half a kilo every week. She was checked every day for signs of self-harm. She lost all sense of herself, she told me. She had no autonomy left at all.

There were fourteen girls on her ward, aged between twelve and seventeen. She would look at the twelve- and thirteen-year-olds and think how sick they were, how young, and then realize that she wasn't much older than them, and she would feel crushed under the weight of that thought.

The girls on her ward were not allowed to go to the toilets unsupervised. They would always be watched. Or, occasionally, if they were doing better, they would be permitted to wee while the nurse stood outside with one foot in the door to keep the girls from slamming it closed. On these days, Rowan was forced to count to ten, loudly, while she was sitting on the toilet, so the nurse could hear each number clear as day. This was, of course, so the girls weren't going to the toilets to throw up, to purge themselves, but Rowan had never done that, she was afraid of vomit, she had only ever withheld, restricted, never taken something into her body and thrown it away again.

There were three tables in the hospital's dining room. The first was for girls who were barely able to swallow solid food and wouldn't eat at all unless there was someone supervising them. They sat under the watchful eye of a nurse who refused to let them leave the table until they had eaten everything on their plate. The second table was for girls who were doing slightly better, who still needed to have their plate checked before going back to their rooms but didn't have to have every mouthful watched, every chew, every swallow. The third table was for the unsupervised girls, the ones on the verge of getting out.

On one particular day, when Rowan was still on the first table, a new nurse arrived in the dining room. She was an agency nurse. Because they weren't permanent staff members in the hospital, agency nurses would come and go from the wards. They often didn't seem to have the kind of training you might expect of a medical professional dealing with such severe mental illness, she tells me. I notice now, as she is speaking, the distance with which she talks about her own mental illness, and I am in awe of how far she has come.

On this day, the agency nurse piled her plate with food but only ate a tiny portion of it. As the nurse went to clear her plate, Rowan said: I don't mean to be rude, but the rule is that everyone, including nurses, must finish everything on their plate within thirty minutes. She had said this after exchanging glances with the other girls on the table, all troubled by the nurse's inability to respect the rules, her dismissal of their needs.

The nurse looked at Rowan and smirked.

If you girls have so much trouble finishing your food, why should I have to?

Then she got up and shovelled the pile of food left on her plate into the bin and walked away. Rowan remembers thinking: What do you think we're doing here?

Rowan says to me: No one with proper training in dealing with severely mentally ill children could be so blasé about their affliction. *If you girls have so much trouble finishing your food, why should I have to?* As though this was a fair fight between this woman and these imprisoned girls.

Because we'll die here if we don't, they thought. Because we are trying to get better. For you it's easy, so show us.

Rowan remembers all sorts of horrifying encounters with agency nurses like this one. But some of the staff were brilliant, she says to me. I genuinely credit them with saving my life.

Rowan had no control over the way her body was changing. It was growing and shifting and it didn't fit her the way it was supposed to.

She couldn't stand being checked for marks, for scars, all the time, and she desperately wanted to be alone in a bathroom, not for any particular reason, just to have the freedom to do it.

The team of doctors did a 'care review' every few weeks to assess each patient's progress. Rowan was aggressively compliant, she told me, she just wanted to get out. But at every care meeting the doctors said she would need another six weeks to recover, and then another, and then another.

I didn't have an unsupervised wee for over five months, she tells me when I ask how long she ended up staying on the ward.

A few months into her stay, Rowan had to rescue a patient, a young woman from her ward who had tried to hang herself outside the door to Rowan's room. With the help of another girl, she cut the rope, screaming until help finally came. The ward was so understaffed that, no matter how well-intentioned the nurses were, they ended up being forced to leave the girls to tend to things they shouldn't have to. She had been living with this girl for three months when this happened. She tells me now that the girl is doing much better.

Sometimes it felt as though the entire hospital was made up only of common areas, Rowan tells me. When girls had incidents like that – this is the word Rowan uses, 'incidents', so mature and wise at nineteen, as if she had spent those months as a trainee nurse rather than a patient – they had them in the hallways.

There is something about this formulation of Rowan's – *when the girls had incidents like that, they had them in the hallways* – that I couldn't let go of, months and months after we spoke. A structure that allows that kind of harm to be on display, allows a person's weakest moments to be witnessed by girls as young as thirteen, feels so cruel. More punishment for the crime of absorbing the messages society sends us.

.   .   .

I think a lot while I am speaking to Rowan about whether I should tell her how severely I have struggled with my own eating disorder. No, strike that: how much I still do.

Is it right to connect yourself with a subject in this way, or is it manipulative? Is it helpful to tell her that I know what it feels like to want to grind yourself into nothingness, or is it harmful?

The day after I speak to Rowan for the first time, I am walking along the Holloway Road towards Highbury and Islington station. It's a walk I do often. I like it and I am a creature of habit. I always have been.

I am listening to a poem by Blythe Baird called 'Relapse'. The poem is about Baird's eating disorder, about falling back into it. It's also about recovery.

These are some of the lines:

> *Last night, I painted my nails when I was hungry.*
> *I can't eat until the polish is dry.*
> *I don't know how to talk about the rabbit hole*
> *without inviting you to follow me down it.*
> *I don't want to go into more detail because what if*
> *you mistake this poem for an instruction manual?*

I don't know how to talk about the rabbit hole without accidentally inviting you to follow me down it. For some reason I am deeply attached to that line. I think about it a lot when I am writing. How can I write a book about all the ways I have struggled to live in my body without it becoming a kind of road map? How do I write about my worst moments without glorifying them? How do I sympathize with Rowan, act like an observer, a conduit for her story, when I am in the grips of the same illness? Do I tell her that I know how it feels? Or is it damaging to her to see someone ten years older who is still stuck in the same pattern? How do I write about her without reconstructing her in the process, without inserting myself into her words?

I do not know the answers to any of these questions. But I am asking them because I am trying to write about lockdown. Which is to say I am trying to write about my own eating disorder, about the way it reared its ugly head again as soon as life threw something at me that I couldn't control. Listening to Rowan's story and seeing myself in it but also feeling somehow disconnected from the version of me who starves herself is a funny kind of cognitive dissonance. I am ashamed of my own shame, and so, too often, I am tempted to bury it.

Growing up as a gymnast meant I was always obsessed with food, but in a relatively healthy way, most of the time. My diet was strictly set by my coaches and I never deviated from it. In some ways, the strict regime was helpful for me. I was always in complete control. I had the most unimaginable willpower because I was so determined to be the best at what I did.

There were bad moments, though, in among it all. The idea that my performance and my ability were so heavily dependent on my body got to me sometimes. To be a nationally competitive gymnast I had to stay as small and muscular as possible, so there were moments when puberty terrified me. Like one day, when I cut a permanent scar into my leg to mark where I could fit my fingers around it, to make sure I would know if my thighs were getting wider.

That loathing brewed inside me for a few years after I quit gymnastics before I started expressing it through disordered eating. I was nineteen when it started, the same age as Rowan is now, speaking so wisely to me about her recovery. I was living in Bristol in the UK because I needed a break from my home town of Sydney. It was a cold winter.

My life didn't have much routine and it was freezing cold outside and it took me a long time to find friends I connected with. So for months, I sat alone in my dorm room watching *Grey's Anatomy* and eating porridge covered in cinnamon for dinner.

On the one day a week I had class on campus, I would stop at Tesco's at the Bristol Triangle and buy share bags of Maltesers, one for every night of the week. I was so lonely, and these rituals comforted me. In a new place, in a new climate, I put on weight quickly.

I have always been very slim, both naturally and because of the obsessive exercise I did growing up. So it might sound silly that someone who is naturally thin could become so destructive around food, so mentally unwell. But body dysmorphia is just that. It lies to you about the way you look and it feeds you a twisted unreality every day until you cannot separate the body in your mind's eye from the body you actually have.

Of course, the body I actually have has important practical impacts, too. The fact that I am thin gives me a degree of privilege I cannot underestimate. It allows me to feel conventionally attractive and allows me to be treated with a kind of sympathy I never would if I had been overweight. Those privileges impact on my life in myriad ways every day, and would have also made my struggle with anorexia easier too. It's important to acknowledge both the power of a disturbed mind to create a trick mirror, and the power of a world that treats you well because of what you look like.

My normal weight is around fifty kilograms. In Bristol, I reached fifty-five kilograms. Every time I looked in the mirror, I felt sick. I couldn't stand how heavy I looked, how round my face had become. I was convinced I looked like I was wearing a fat suit, like Gwyneth Paltrow in Shallow Hal.

At first, I just exercised obsessively. I started running every day and doing as many exercise classes at the gym as I could possibly manage.

I love exercise; it makes me feel powerful and alive. It was easy to convince myself that addiction to it was healthy. Addiction is never healthy; I know that now.

I finally settled into my new town and made some friends I would keep for the next nine years. I slowly grew happier, and I let the obsession slide.

But then my semester was up, and I had to come home. Back in Sydney, I felt out of control all over again. I had decided to leave because I needed everything about my life to change. I had come out of a very bad break-up that I couldn't move on from and nothing in my life made sense to me. I also developed my first bouts of what would become lifelong chronic pain and illness. I hated being sick, and Sydney was where I had first got sick. I couldn't stand it there.

What I now know, looking back on this time, is that I was also developing my first symptoms of post-traumatic stress disorder as a result of my rape. My mental health was crumbling and I couldn't think my way out of it. So I did what I had always done: I ran away.

·   ·   ·

Rowan is beautiful and healthy-looking when I speak to her, just a few short years after she was discharged from the ward. She has long, flowing dark hair that is lighter at the bottom, and a fringe that sits wistfully across her face. She sips bubble tea and smiles constantly, a genuine smile, one that warms me from the inside out.

Rowan was stuck in hospital for most of the second half of her GCSE year, so she had to revise on the ward. She was forced to drop all sciences because her teachers said it was too hard to teach her physics and chemistry remotely.

Whenever she had time to herself on the ward, Rowan studied. She had always been stubborn as hell, she told me, and the exams were a way of reminding herself that the outside world was still out there, that if she kept putting on weight and playing by the rules she could be out in time to sit her exams with the rest of her school.

She knew she wanted to study English and creative writing at university, and one of the nurses had been a high school English teacher before he returned to study to become a nurse. So every day when making sure she had no self-inflicted wounds, or escorting her for every weigh-in, or taking her blood pressure, he would talk to her about the books she was studying. He helped her understand the texts and he would talk to her for as long as she needed, and it really helped her. She also found a French-speaking staff member on a nearby ward who would help her practise for her French GCSE. She worked so hard, knowing that she would be out by the time of her exams.

But she wasn't. Rowan was transported from the hospital ward to her old high school to sit her exams, and then transported back when they were over. Still, some way, somehow, she passed every single one. Isn't that remarkable? I think that's remarkable. I gasp when she tells me this during our interview.

Her response is very different to mine. She says: Because I knew if I passed my exams they would let me out of there. I knew it would convince them I was well.

I am in awe at her determination. But I also understand it. I've been there in some sense. I've been on the bathroom floor, sick and convulsing with pain, thinking: I'll do whatever it takes to make this stop. I'll do anything. Watch me.

. . .

When Rowan speaks, I am thinking about how this is also connected to the way we are personally blamed for the consequences of intense structural pressure to perfect our bodies. Society makes us ashamed of ourselves and our physical forms, so, in order to survive, we change them. But then we are blamed for our self-inflicted wounds, for the damage we cause ourselves. But it isn't us. It's them. The determination is part of proving this, at least for me. It's a way of saying: Look how far I will go to recover. Let me prove I did not choose this. I did not want this, I was born into it. You call this self-harm to clear your own conscience, but we all know it isn't.

. . .

When I speak to Rowan now, she says that the voices in her head are still there. The ones that convince her if she breathes too close to her housemates' dinner plates, the calories might absorb straight through her nose and into her blood. The ones that have memorized the calorie count of every major food item. But she is getting better at ignoring the voices, she tells me, and eating the food anyway. It is a daily battle, but it is one she is winning.

It was the girls on the ward who got her through, Rowan says, that's the truth of it. She would never have become free – either physically or psychologically – if it wasn't for them. There was a group of about six of them who became very, very close. All they wanted for each other was for each of them to get better, to see what friendship felt like on the outside. It's funny that my own experience of teenage girl-friendship seemed so defined by competition – perhaps it was the athlete in me, the ghost of the gymnastics floor in every social interaction. The need to prove I could win. In a different circumstance, in a different world, it was made of allyship. It's a strange privilege to have, to fall out with friends over boys and parties rather than bond over terrible wards and uncomfortable examinations, but it is a privilege nonetheless.

They confided in each other and counted down the days to each weekly yoga class in a room downstairs from the ward. The external yoga teacher treated them like girls, Rowan tells me, not patients. It was the only time in the week they could pretend they might be able to all go to brunch together afterwards and talk about normal, teenage girl things.

Rowan was released from hospital just over five months after she arrived. She went home to her parents' house, went back to school, back to normal life as best she could. She passed her A levels and was accepted to university to study English literature and creative writing. Just before she started university, she met up with her best friend from the ward. They were both on the outside now, and they walked together along London's South Bank and had a drink together on a rooftop under the summer sun. She was seventeen.

· · ·

I was the age Rowan is now when I first got properly sick when it came to eating. I think about her now, so poised, and about how she is already out the other side of a battle I had only just begun. What does that mean about how things have changed, I wonder. Are things getting worse instead of better? Is there even more pressure to promote the lie that we are thinner, better, than we are? Or are there better mediums for it?

Just after my nineteenth birthday, I stopped going out because I couldn't stand the way I looked in my clothes. I had a lecture that semester with an ex-boyfriend and I couldn't stand the thought that he saw me every day in my new form. I started digging my thumbs into my wrists before and after that lecture, so the marks would remind me later how bad it had felt and would stop me from eating. It didn't work. I kept eating every mealtime and hating myself for it. I started throwing up my food twice a day – once in the morning, with the shower running, and once at night-time, when my housemates were asleep.

Eventually I signed up with a personal trainer and he taught me how to avoid carbs in my diet and how to exercise to lose weight. Once I had a set of rules, it was easy. I just followed them obsessively. I have always been good like this. I lost twelve kilos this way. By the time my parents intervened and asked me if I had an eating disorder, I weighed forty-three kilograms and was 165 centimetres tall.

When I met Rowan, I had just come back from my first book tour. I travelled to Australia and did events about *I Choose Elena* in Sydney, Melbourne, Brisbane and Adelaide.

I don't know if it was the publicity or the constant talk about my own sense of unworthiness, but the tour brought my aesthetic self-hate back like I had never imagined, and the eating problems came soon after. I started obsessing over how large I looked in pictures of myself at events and on television. I sat for hours poring over video footage of my TV appearance trying to catch myself at a different angle to prove I was slimmer than I looked, but it didn't work. My body stayed the same at every angle. So I had to change it.

As I write this, the government has allowed us only one trip outdoors each day to exercise. It is only supposed to be sixty minutes long, but every morning I wake up, drink a glass of sparkling water with a squeeze of lemon juice – if taken first thing, it speeds up the metabolism – and run for at least an hour and a half, meditating the whole time on how big my thighs look in my jogging pants and how much better I'll feel when I am slim again. I count calories every day and I keep a meticulous food diary and I exercise pathologically in my bedroom and I waste hours scrolling through photos of Instagram models I want to look like.

I am a high-risk patient for coronavirus – I have two chronic illness and I take immunosuppressants every day. If I contract this virus, I am among the most likely group of people to develop severe complications. I could die. And yet I am flouting government advice by staying out of doors longer than I am supposed to because I am so desperate to lose weight. I am risking contracting a disease that could kill me in order to feed another disease that could kill me. I am sick.

How did I get here? How could it be that I have published a book about exorcizing my demons when in truth I have done nothing of the sort? How could I have looked squarely at my sense of unworthiness and wholly failed to remove this piece of it? How could I have been sitting in Emma's living room a few months earlier, wondering how to intervene to protect her slim thirteen-year-old body from herself when I can't even protect my own?

.   .   .

I think about this as I slowly piece together the story of Rachel, a woman I interviewed for this book. She said she wanted to tell me about getting trapped in an abusive intimate relationship that she thought was about her experience of sex, but to explain that, she said, she had to take me back even further.

.   .   .

When Rachel was nine, her grandfather stopped coming over to visit. This devastated her, because Rachel and her grandfather were extraordinarily close. She kept asking her mother what had happened, but she never got a clear answer. She was being treated like a child, but she knew something was very wrong.

A few years later, her mother finally told her that she had cut off contact with her grandfather after it came out that he had sexually abused her aunt – her mother's sister – when she was a child. This was shocking news to a not-yet-teenage Rachel, who adored her grandfather. But then her mother said to her, Don't worry, I have never left you alone with him.

But that wasn't true, Rachel thought. She had often been alone with him as a child. She knew that nothing terrible had ever happened, but she also knew she had memories of him being inappropriate with her. She remembers being bounced on his crotch in a way she did not like. She had always known these memories were uncomfortable, but they became very menacing when she received this news about her grandfather being an abuser. She would find out later that he had physically abused her cousins and aunts and uncles as well.

Rachel kept seeing her grandfather for supervised visits because she missed him terribly, but she also knew that something felt like it had shifted in her.

A few years later, Rachel was having a difficult time in high school. She had felt self-loathing creep up on her as she grew into adolescence. She started cutting deep ridges into her wrists until she was called into the principal's office to try and address the issue.

But one of the teachers standing in the room said to the principal: They are just little scratches. She's just being attention-seeking.

Rachel laughs a bit as she tells me this story, as she says: Of course the first thing I did when I got home was to make sure I cut deeper next time. I took it as a challenge.

This makes me think about how often we are gaslighted, disbelieved, belittled, that by fourteen years old we know that even our desire to self-destruct requires a heavy burden of proof.

Rachel went home and cut herself more, and more, and more, hoping the teachers would take her seriously, but they did not.

The next year, Rachel started feeling even worse about herself and her body. She was feeling confused about her sexuality and confused about what she wanted to look like. And so she did the thing so many of us do when we want our borders to soften and dissolve, when we wish desperately not to be seen. She stopped eating.

But the same thing happened again. When Rachel took herself to her GP to ask for help, to say she had an eating disorder, the doctor said: Your cheeks are too round for you to be anorexic.

Deflated, feeling as though she had failed again, failed at starving herself, failed at convincing the doctor she was credible, failed at being desperate enough to deserve help, she went home and allowed the eating disorder to swallow her whole, determined to be successful next time around.

. . .

This part of Rachel's story breaks my heart, and it makes me think a lot of myself when I was that age. I desperately wanted someone to notice that I was unwell, that I wasn't eating, that I was hurting myself. I didn't want to say the words, so I let it show up on my body instead, hoping that someone would notice, but no one did.

This gets me thinking about the cruel double bind of the phrase 'attention-seeking' when levelled at women, especially young women and girls. It has been contorted into an accusation, something shameful. But in reality, it isn't. Of course Rachel was being attention-seeking. So was Rowan. So was Emma. So was I. In a world that wouldn't listen when we spoke, we were trying to use whatever method we could to scream for intervention. We were being attention-seeking because no one was paying attention, and we desperately needed them to. We were screaming *help me*. Where is the moral failure in that?

Another moment from my childhood comes to mind. I was fifteen, and I was writing a short story for a secondary school fiction prize. I told my English tutor that I would like to write about disordered eating.

No, no way, my tutor said. Sorry, she added when she saw my face fall.

Why not? I asked.

Because the judges won't even read it. They will toss away any stories that deal with silly teenage girl topics. They'll see it as attention-seeking.

The idea didn't sit well with me even then, but I quickly assessed that there was not much I could do about it.

Now I think about how strange this was. Write what you know, they always tell us. *Write what you know.* But if you're a teenage girl, it's not so straightforward.

Write what you know, they say.

But oh no, not that, they qualify. Oh, not that either. Or that.

Maybe don't write.

I remember how pervasive this idea was in high school: that girlhood was an exaggeration, a red herring. That we amplified our pain instead of metabolizing it. But that was never true, even then. Especially then. We spent so much more energy hiding our suffering than we did voicing it, and they still called us liars.

CHAPTER FOUR

What I learned from the interviews I did for this book is that to know you are one thing and be told you are another is a singular form of shame transmission. It is the same thing I keep coming back to, again and again, in these interviews: it is the horror of not knowing what is real and what isn't, of being taught not to trust yourself, of never knowing who to believe, of knowing your own reality won't be trusted if you dare to speak it aloud.

It is wearing the scars of a life spent fighting to be seen and understood and recognized and believed. It is constantly battling against voices telling you that you are not valid or honest or real.

The non-binary writer Alok Vaid-Menon describes this in their book, *Beyond the Gender Binary*. Like everything in these interviews, it seems to all come down to one thing. Shame.

'The thing about shame is that it eats at you until it fully consumes you. Then you cannot tell the difference between their shame and your own – between a body and an apology,' Vaid-Menon writes. 'It's not just that you internalize the shame; rather, it becomes you. You no longer need the people at school telling you not to dress like that; you already do it to yourself.'

It's not just that you internalize shame; rather, it becomes you.

Shame is born out of the idea that there is a particular order to the universe that we must accede to if we are to live. It tells us there is a group armed with accepted wisdom that has the power to exclude us.

Shame is a truly deadly emotion. It is pure evil. It is a liar. It is the emotion that supports and breathes life into every form of structural oppression we have ever created. It is the way that systemic unfairness gets under our skin and into our blood and bones.

It is so powerful that we are never taught to question its authority. Writing this book, it strikes me that perhaps that's what true power is: the structural and systemic privilege of being allowed to define what is normal and what is abnormal, what is acceptable and what is shameful, what is allowed to be flaunted and what is to be kept secret.

Another thing I kept coming back to in the interviews I did for this book is that there is an intense and powerful connection between shame and language. One of the most important gatekeepers of shame is our determination not to give people the words they need to speak freely about themselves.

This was certainly true of my rape and my trauma. For eleven years, I did not have the words to speak about what had happened to me because no one around me was speaking about it. There were no words that were good enough.

Shame lives and breathes in silence. When we make people ashamed, we both create and recreate that prison by ensuring that it cannot be spoken about.

This is something I heard again and again from the non-binary people I spoke to about this book. They had lived their whole lives knowing the truth about themselves, knowing that their bodies didn't fit them the way they were supposed to, knowing that they felt uncomfortable in their own skin because of how society reflected their identity back at them.

So many people misinterpret gender-fluidity or dysmorphia as confusion, but none of the people I spoke to recall ever feeling confused. They always knew the truth, they just didn't have the words.

As Bernardine Evaristo writes in *Girl, Woman, Other*, being gender-queer, trans or gender-fluid 'wasn't about playacting an identity on a whim, it's about becoming your true self in spite of society's pressures to be otherwise'.

Everyone I spoke to for this book said they were relieved when they first heard the term non-binary. They knew immediately that's what they were. For each person I spoke to, this realization came when they connected, often by chance or by the grace of the internet, with a queer community big enough to include other non-binary people. Those non-binary friends would introduce them to the concept and explain what it meant, what it felt like, and they would know they had found the right word, the right signifier, to speak their truth to the world.

This taught me two things that I already suspected about bodies and shame. The first thing is that language is how we crawl out from underneath shame. The second is that human connection and empathy – the enemies of shame – are crucial to learning the language we need to define ourselves.

Neither alone is sufficient, but both are necessary. The writer Maggie Nelson asks, in *The Argonauts*, her own memoir about loving her partner, a trans man: 'Are words good enough?' Perhaps the answer is yes, but only when they are paired with love.

In 'The Struggles of Rejecting the Gender Binary', a piece in the *New York Times*, non-binary specialist therapist Jan Tate describes treating Salem, a non-binary patient in the process of coming out.

Tate said, 'I often find myself gut-knotted after sessions with Salem, because of the things they don't say' – because of the feelings Salem kept locked away, even from her, for fear that their experience was inexpressible, incomprehensible.

In this same article, Salem says something to the journalist that also accords with everything I have learned over the last few years about bodies and shame: 'One of the hardest things for me is to say to myself, Yes, I'm real.'

Yes, I'm real.

When Salem talks to the journalist about coming out, about learning to inhabit their body, they refer to the book-turned-film *Into the Wild*, where the main character dies of starvation in the wildness, not knowing that he is only half a mile from safety, that if he walked a little bit further, he would find relief.

'People say the dude was an idiot,' Salem said to Tate, 'because he could have lived if he realized there was a crossing nearby. But I can understand him. To me, he's relatable.'

It was as if Salem both knew and didn't know that other places existed, the journalist wrote.

A study by Pace, a mental health charity for lesbian, gay, bisexual and transgender people, in partnership with Brunel University, the University of Worcester and London South Bank University, found that 59% of trans people under twenty-six had considered attempting suicide, 48% had actually attempted it, and 30% of respondents had attempted suicide in the past year.

A peer-reviewed study published by the *Journal of Adolescent Health* in 2020, 'Understanding the Mental Health of Transgender and Nonbinary Youth', which includes data from 25,000 queer young people between the ages of thirteen and twenty-four, found that a third of non-binary children and young people had attempted suicide in the last twelve months.

Most non-Western cultures have deeply established concepts of gender-fluidity and concepts of gender that are much broader than the binary. Since antiquity, India has had a vibrant transgender culture, known as hijras, and recently decided to appoint a new transgender deity to worship. The Supreme Court in Pakistan recognizes the third gender on national identity cards. The Indonesian Bugis ethnic group recognizes five genders. South Asian religious traditions honour people who are 'sacred mediators between males and females and between the spheres of humans and the domain of spirits', as noted in Michael G. Peletz's book *Gender Pluralism: Southeast Asia Since Early Modern Times*.

The gender binary is a wholly Western construct. It is not real. It is a structure built by Westerners, maintained by Western culture.

As Salem told the *New York Times*, we are all born non-binary. Gender is the thing that is false. Gender is learned.

Not long after I speak to Rowan, I meet Jules, who is twenty-three now and has just come out as non-binary and has started to use they/ them pronouns. We speak over Zoom and I am immediately captivated by them.

They have a brilliantly wide smile and an energetic tone that makes me feel immediately connected to them. They have an American accent but I know from our email conversations arranging the interview that they live in Brussels, so I am intrigued. We are on different continents, but I feel immediately as though we are in the same room.

Jules' parents are both American, originally from San Francisco, but they met in Germany in the 1950s and moved to Brussels together after they married. After twenty years of raising their children in Brussels, they moved back to the States in the early 2010s.

Jules tells me they always liked Brussels growing up, but when they were a teenager it started to feel small and stifling. They started to feel as though they didn't quite fit in with their friends, either their German-speaking friends or their English-speaking ones. Brussels felt a lot like a small town in some ways. Everyone went to the same restaurants, the same shopping malls, the same bars. It was hard to find a new crowd.

Jules found themself without anyone to talk to about their sexuality when they started wondering whether they were straight. All their friends started dating boys, and Jules did too, but they were never totally taken with the idea. They started to feel more and more alone as high school wore on, and eventually they decided that the best thing to do as soon as they could would be to move away.

Knowing they wanted to study English and creative writing, Jules applied to universities all over Europe. With fluency in both English and German, they weren't short of options, and they had always done well in school. Jules chose Leeds University.

Not knowing what to expect, Jules packed up their things in their childhood bedroom and thought about Yorkshire. They had never even been there before, and it felt good to be taking a leap into the unknown. I nod when they tell me this. I know that feeling.

The day they arrived was blustery, cold and overcast – something they would come to realize is not unusual for Leeds in September. But they felt optimistic.

The world seemed to open up to Jules as they started classes. They liked their professors and their classmates. Eventually they would grow discontented with the degree itself, but they liked being there enough to stick it out for a couple of years.

One of their best friends from halls started taking them to cool, alternative bars around town and introducing them to her gay friends.

I need to introduce you to every single one of them, the friend said.

Why? Jules asked her.

Because you are so gay, their friend said, and laughed. Jules laughed too, and thought that their friend might be on to something, they tell me now.

Over the two years that followed, Jules was finally able to embrace their sexuality fully. The queer community in Leeds was like nothing they had ever experienced before – certainly nothing like what was on offer in Brussels. The more people they met in the sprawling group of gay friends they had adopted, the more at home they felt. They got their first girlfriend at the end of the first year. The two of them fell in love quickly and slowly at the same time, switching between diving in and holding back.

Inside that relationship, Jules was able to properly experience queer sex for the first time. They loved the way they could be intimate with their girlfriend and explore non-heteronormative closeness and pleasure. In a lot of ways, they felt like the two of them grew up together.

They broke up the following May, around exam time, but it was amicable and sweet. They both needed to move on. Jules' friends joked about how they would have to adjust to the queer break-up – no space, no ghosting, an immediate shift into close friendship, because they were all committed to loving each other no matter what, and because they all needed each other, too.

After the break-up, Jules became more and more disillusioned with university but more and more enamoured with their community. They swapped studying for nights out at fringe comedy clubs and queer collective spaces. They met a couple of friends who had exactly the same aesthetic as them – androgynous, thin, jackets, glasses, patches, boots. They described themselves as non-binary, which was a term Jules had not heard before.

They talked about not feeling at home with a female body or identity. They talked about not wanting to identify as men either. Transition didn't feel right. Staying in their own bodies didn't feel right either.

This is exactly how Jules had felt since high school – an uncomfortable sense of things not fitting. They were so inspired by the non-binary folks they met, loved their confidence, their radiance, their self-assuredness. As soon as they saw this feeling expressed in a living, breathing body, they knew they wanted to express it too.

.   .   .

The first time I read *The Argonauts* by Maggie Nelson, I was sitting in my bedroom in my home town of Sydney, Australia. It is a memoir about a relationship, it is literary criticism, it is gender theory, queer theory, ontology, it is specific and universal, creative and critical. Nelson says that her partner Harry, a trans man in the throes of hormone treatment, asked her, 'What's your pleasure?' and then 'stuck around for an answer'.

So she sends him a passage from Roland Barthes, one that explains that saying 'I love you' is like 'the Argonaut renewing his ship during its voyage without changing its name'. The name – the words – are the same, but the meaning of them is remade every time they are spoken. Two pages later, Nelson quotes Barthes: 'the very task of love and of language is to give to one and the same phrase inflections which will be forever new.' She makes this point again later in the book when she tells us: 'Words change depending on who speaks them.'

But the truth of this book comes crashing in on the page after this, when Nelson reflects on Harry's response to the Barthes offering: 'I thought the passage was romantic,' Nelson writes. 'You read it as a possible retraction. In retrospect, I guess it was both.'

I guess it was both.

Nelson starts *The Argonauts* by asking whether words are good enough. She asks this question again and again. She says she has spent a lifetime devoted to Wittgenstein's notion that the inexpressible is contained – inexpressibly! – in the expressed. 'Its paradox is, quite literally, why I write, or how I feel able to keep writing,' Nelson tells us.

By the second or third reading of this book, I realized this is why I write, too. Like all the best writers, Nelson was explaining something to me that I knew, but which was too fundamental to be expressible, at least by me.

Words are good enough, Nelson insists. Because even though there are things they cannot contain, even though there are things we cannot say, every time we sit down to try, we circle closer to making those slippery things expressible.

But Harry disagrees. Harry believes that once you put something into words, you imprison it. That you murder something by defining it. Which of them is right? Maybe both. Maybe it's a question that we can keep coming back to, again and again. Maybe that's what real love – the kind Nelson and Harry have – is all about. It's the same as her love for writing. It's the same as mine. The very task of love and of language is to give to one and the same phrase inflections which will be forever new.

As a way – I like to think – of answering Harry's question ('What's your pleasure?'), Nelson writes:

The pleasure of recognizing that one may have to undergo the same realizations, write the same notes in the margin, return to the same themes in one's work, relearn the same emotional truths, write the same book over and over again.

As Nelson tells the story of her life with Harry – of his journey through hormone treatment and transition, of her journey through pregnancy and birth and motherhood – she shows us the kind of devotion that constitutes a life. In doing that, she gives us something we can revisit, again and again, and find something new in each time. In her ordinary devotion to writing, in her determination to find the inexpressible in the expressed, she proves the theory she has set out to test. Words are different depending on who speaks – or reads – them.

And that's what this book taught me: that love does not have to mean believing wholly in something. Love does not mean the absence of doubt. Love means knowing that sometimes words don't work, but we keep trying anyway, because we know that we get closer each time we try. Love means believing in the process and sitting in the uncertainty of the outcome. Are words good enough, or not good enough? I guess it is both.

Unflinching and beautiful. Doubt and devotion. Theory and memoir. Inexpressible and – somehow – expressed. Feral with vulnerability and steady with courage. Humbled by words but brave with them. Humbled by love but brave with it.

Each time I read this book, I learn something new about love. Which is to say I learn something new about writing. Which is to say that this book refuses to be bounded, refuses to be one thing, refuses to shy away from the uncertainty of love and vulnerability and doubt. That's the most important thing a writer can do. Maggie Nelson taught me that – again and again.

I am thinking about *The Argonauts* a lot after my interview with Jules. The idea of finding a new language to hold your experiences in is, it seems to me, one of the cornerstones of freedom. Finding words that are good enough. They and them and non-binary and genderqueer and trans-masculine and assigned female at birth.

.　　　.　　　.

I am still thinking about Maggie Nelson when I meet Pat. Pat is small, and blonde, and works as a computer technician in London.

When Pat was very small, they asked their parents to call them Boris. They don't remember exactly why they chose Boris, but we both laugh at this bold choice when they tell me.

Pat was assigned female at birth but they always knew they were not a 'real' girl. Those are the first terms they remember thinking about it in. Not a real girl. Something else, but they didn't know what. They didn't think they were a boy either.

This feeling was all right in the first ten or so years of their life. It didn't bother them too much. They resisted any girly nicknames or outfits and their parents embraced and respected this completely.

But then I hit puberty, they tell me, and my body turned into a girl's body, and I couldn't stand it. I hated the way it looked and felt and the way it was growing.

Pat didn't develop an interest in having boyfriends or girlfriends when all their friends did. They remember just thinking: I guess that's not for me. Their only relationship to their body was that they hated it aesthetically, and they had no concept of it functionally because they had no interest in sex or relationships.

Everyone around Pat – their friends at school, their parents – assumed this was because they were gay and only wanted to date women. One day, they came home from school and their parents had left a leaflet on the table that they had ordered from the Stonewall charity: HOW TO TALK TO YOUR CHILD ABOUT BEING GAY, it said.

Look! Pat's mother said. I have this and I read it, let's talk.

It was just the sweetest thing, Pat says to me now as they recall it in our interview.

But Pat didn't think they were gay.

I didn't think I was anything, they say to me. I was just, nothing.

This chimes with something I have heard so often while writing this book: It just felt like I wasn't real, like I had never existed, like maybe I wasn't really there.

As high school wore on, Pat started to think they were bisexual, because they felt drawn to both men and women but not to either gender in particular.

I never came out as bisexual, because it seemed so obvious to me, Pat told me. Nothing about the idea of an either/or question ever made sense to me when it came to gender or sexuality, so categorizing myself as straight or gay never felt right either.

When they realized they were bisexual, Pat thought this was the label they needed in order to demystify their identity. To feel real.

I thought: Okay, great, that's what I am, they say to me in 2020. Pat is soft-spoken and I am captivated by them.

.   .   .

I meet Ingrid on Twitter and we speak at length about their experience of living outside the gender binary, their experience of coming out. The stories they tell me, which I will recreate here, feel so powerful to me. Their descriptions of never feeling at home in their own flesh. Ingrid is twenty-two when we speak, but they take me back to their teenage years to tell me this story.

Ingrid woke up early and showered slowly, thinking about the left-over pieces of a dream they'd had, something about a girl they knew in primary school. It was freezing outside and their boiler was broken again. They knew this the minute they swam into consciousness.

Their body was stiff and rigid under the duvet, bracing itself against the cold. They shuddered as they threw off the covers, cursing the strange and mysterious machine that was supposed to keep the house warm. Their feet fell heavily on the lacquered floor in the hallway. The wood felt near frozen. They thought about how strange it is that in the first few seconds of touching something very hot or very cold, sometimes the two sensations feel the same. The bathroom door creaked as they opened it. The bones in their wrists creaked too, full of dust. When they stepped out of the shower they pulled on their swimming costume and looked at their shoulders. They were strong and broad, which they liked.

They crossed their arms across their chest and held onto each shoulder, pressing their fingers into their knotted muscles, enjoying how tactile those shoulders were. They stood like this for a full five minutes, staring at themself as they massaged their shoulders, feeling calm. They looked out of the window. It was snowing again.

Ingrid felt at home in water. Here, their body felt at rest. At swimming practice that morning, they were energized. They swam front crawl faster than usual and their coach was pleased. They had a big competition coming up that weekend, the regional championships for under-fifteens.

Still smelling of chlorine, they pulled on their school uniform. Their legs and shoulders ached. They were dreading the day. But they were doing English first thing, which was their favourite subject. The thought of reading relaxed them, like water.

At break time, they found their group of friends standing by the water fountains, yelling raucously about something. One of the boys – and they were all boys except Ingrid – wanted to change the rules of their daily handball tournament to include a sudden death round at the end of lunch. This would mean players would be eliminated after one mess-up, which was a very controversial suggestion.

The handball game was already a high-stakes endeavour. It was the thing they all looked forward to most. Losing status or falling behind in the handball rankings – which were etched in chalk on the wall next to the metal seats that demarcated this group's spot – was devastating. Especially for Ingrid, who had to work every day to convince themself they were allowed to be part of this group of boys. They wondered how they would fare in a sudden death situation.

The boys yelled at each other for the rest of break time and eventually the pro-sudden-death faction won out. As they walked back to class, Ingrid asked one of the boys in their swim team why he had missed practice that morning. He was a dedicated swimmer, like Ingrid, and they were surprised he would miss training so close to competition day. He looked at Ingrid guiltily as he said he'd slept in, he'd stayed up too late playing World of Warcraft. They laughed and rolled their eyes.

As they pushed open the door of their house, Ingrid could tell the boiler was still broken. It was cold, even for November. Even for the Midlands. Even for this little house, in this village. They shuddered as they thought about waking up the next morning to swim.

Their mother was fussing in their bedroom when they walked in. They hated it when their mother did this. They wished she would give them some privacy. She had started taking offence when Ingrid chose to hide their body from her when they were getting changed.

Her mother was moving things around on their desk.

Hi, Mum, Ingrid said.

Hi, darling. Her tone was clipped. How was school?

Fine. Good, actually. I won handball at lunch. In a sudden death round.

Their mother said nothing, just continued pottering. They sensed the shadow of a 'tut' that almost escaped their mother's lips. They withdrew.

Their mother was folding their clothes now, hastily, as if eager to leave the room now Ingrid was in it. She held up a pair of Ingrid's shorts.

Why do you dress like this, love? she asked.

Ingrid shrugged.

Why don't we go shopping for some nice skirts, now that you're about to start high school? Or some dresses?

Ingrid shrugged again.

Don't you want to wear dresses like the other girls?

Not really.

Why not?

Because I feel strange in dresses. I don't like them.

Why not?

I just don't like them.

I just think you'll have an easier time at your new school if you don't dress like such a tomboy.

Okay. Maybe. I'll think about it.

Great. How was swimming practice this morning?

Good. I was fast.

Good.

Their mother finished folding the clothes in silence. Ingrid watched, breathing her in.

Ingrid started having sex with men at fifteen even though they didn't want to, and this experience – this entering and re-entering vulnerability they never wanted, one which terrified them – left them feeling in their early teens like they didn't have a body at all, Ingrid tells me. They were a floating head.

They would dress up like a 1950s housewife on the weekends because they wanted to be feminine but didn't know how, so they started copying the Audrey Hepburn posters on the walls of their mother's house. They needed a way to be, they tell me. I just needed a way to be.

By the time they were fourteen they were so consumed by their friends' pursuit of boys, so underexposed to anything else in their Midlands town, that they figured if they participated in it long enough, they would like it too. That their eyes would flash when a boy sent a Snapchat asking them to go to the movies, the way their female friends' did. Ingrid figured it was like drinking coffee, or wine. An acquired taste. They stuck with it.

When I ask them how long they did this for, they tell me it must have been years. They knew something was wrong because they never felt at ease around men, and their body burned from the inside out every time they had sex, and they felt uncomfortable talking about sex and thinking about sex and even listening to other people talk about it. I know this feeling, I think as they tell me this last part.

Ingrid is autistic, and as a teenager most social interactions were strained for them anyway, so they thought this was just a harder version of the life they were condemned to. Because no one was around to help them understand their autism, they tell me, they didn't know where it began and ended, and so they didn't know they were queer and non-binary until years later.

Ingrid moved through their adolescence in someone else's life, in someone else's body. They knew that their life didn't fit them the way it was supposed to, but they didn't know what to do about it, didn't know how to blow it up and start again, so they tinkered around the edges. They knew they wanted to look more masculine so they avoided the oral contraceptive pill because it famously gives new life to breasts and hips, parts of themself they wanted to erase. This left them in a constant state of anxiety about pregnancy: a terrible consequence of a terrible life, and a terrible end to a story they never wanted.

When they started university and moved away from the small village near Birmingham where they had grown up and where they had always lived, they felt frozen with fear at the idea of meeting new people. Their physical form was so alien to them, and yet it was the one they would be forced to present themself in. This seemed, to them, a conundrum. They hadn't started dressing in men's clothing yet, so they were a body they didn't recognize wrapped in clothing they had copied from an Audrey Hepburn poster. They hated every inch of it.

So they tell me about how they did the only thing they could think to do: they tried to diminish it as much as they could. They stopped eating, started throwing up half their meals. Gave themself a goal weight to reach by Freshers' week. Thought of little else all year. Just focused on getting smaller and smaller until everything about them stopped feeling so heavy and wrong. By the time they got to university they had lost a stone.

.   .   .

I think of Emma then, of how the two of them are separated by over a decade and half the country, about how different their lives are to one another's, about how they will never meet, but they are similar in this one, specific, ghostly endeavour.

.   .   .

Ingrid is twenty-two by the time I meet them, and they are finally starting to feel comfortable being gender non-conforming, they tell me. Yesterday, they say, they went shopping in the men's section of Topshop in their small country town, and, just for a moment, they didn't even mind who saw them.

.   .   .

A few weeks later, I speak to Jules again. We pick up where we left off: in Leeds.

The more Jules learned about their new friends, the more they admired them. They were confident and authentic and embracing their identity, and they were so happy. Their smiles were so genuine, Jules said to me.

And the more I loved them and looked up to them, the more I realized how contradictory that was, they say, and I nod.

I could see in them all the things I hated about myself, but as soon as they were external to me, I could see their value.

In this one comment, Jules strikes on something that I found in almost every single interview I did for this book. We are taught for so long to dislike ourselves that we can only approve of our own humanity when it is reflected back through someone else. So many women and non-binary people told me a similar story: they had people in their lives that they looked up to, that they thought were beautiful and assured and real, but they couldn't see that they had qualities worthy of that admiration too; they could only see their own qualities in a positive light when they saw them reflected in someone else.

What does that mean about how we are taught to feel about ourselves, I think. I had this exact experience with one of my best friends growing up. I adored her so completely, was so jealous of her, even though her life was very similar to my own. She was the unattainable love object, and so was I, somehow. I am bisexual and I have had many relationships with women, so I don't know if I was in love with her or infatuated with her or just using her as a mirror.

There is something fundamental in this, some truth about womanhood, about the self and the other, about shame and self-destruction and self-harm, about how liking ourselves is so antithetical to what women have been taught that it has to be rerouted through the other qualities they have been erroneously taught are intrinsic to womanhood: jealousy and competition.

In a group of women, this creates a peculiar pattern. Each one is the object of another's admiration, but is, in all likelihood, as uncomfortable in her own skin as the admirer is in theirs. This round robin means that every person is the subject of admiration, but not the object, and is never able to give this admiration to themselves.

When Jules realized how much they were looking up to their friends' gender-fluidity and unapologetic expression, they started trying to turn that gaze on themself. They started talking to their friends about non-binary identity and the support they received was overwhelming. It filled them up.

At around the same time, though, Jules had to admit that they wanted to leave university. They were truly sick of reading boring white male authors who had nothing to recommend them except their status in a literary canon Jules did not see as valid. Their studies were getting more and more difficult to bear. They felt the best thing to do was to leave and move back to Brussels, because it was the place they knew best, even though they didn't much like it, to try and find a different way into the literary world.

·　　·　　·

Pat didn't start experimenting with sex or intimacy until they arrived at university, either.

Their first partner was assigned male at birth and, while the two were together, presented as male. But she confided in Pat that she felt like a woman, and slowly asked Pat to treat her like a woman in bed. Between them, they came up with an amazingly dynamic sexual existence, Pat tells me. I liked that she was fluid and exploring, because it meant that I could be, too. We discovered so many things together.

Plus, Pat says, when you're having queer and gender-fluid sex, you have to talk about things constantly and always communicate, because it's harder to work out what to do. I loved that part of it, Pat said.

Pat's first partner has transitioned since then, and she and Pat and Pat's current partner are all still close friends.

Having my first sexual experience be with a trans person was really life-changing, Pat says to me.

Pat met their current partner not long after, and they have now been together for five years. When I interview Pat over Zoom, they have just moved into a house the two of them bought together. They are at that stage where they are still eating meals on the floor or balanced precariously on top of empty cardboard boxes in lieu of real furniture. Pat seems so happy when they tell me this, and I feel so happy for them.

It wasn't until about a year ago that Pat formally came out as non-binary, to their partner, their parents and their friends.

All of our friends are LGBTQ-aligned in some way, Pat says to me, and soon I started meeting people who identified as non-binary. I'd never heard the term before, they tell me, but I knew immediately: that's what I am. That's what I've always been.

They felt so relieved to have found a word, a label, that encapsulated their not-girl-ness in a way that didn't mean they had to identify strictly as male. They had found a word to wrap themself comfortably inside, and it felt like coming home.

When Jules and I speak they are sitting in their apartment in Brussels and have just helped a housemate move some new furniture into their shared living space. They have also recently come out to all their friends and family as non-binary.

Jules' struggle with their gender identity and the tumult of their early twenties took a toll on their mental health. During those last months in England, they hated their body so much, hated the way it felt and moved and looked, hated that they didn't know what to do about it. So, like so many young people in this book, they took control in one of the only ways they could: they stopped eating.

While struggling to keep up with a degree that had stopped making sense to them and while battling their deteriorating mental health, they started restricting what they put in their body, desperate to make themself smaller, wanting to disappear into thin air. As they ate less and less, their energy plummeted and their mood dropped even further. First they cut out carbs, then fat, until they were eating almost nothing. They tell me you could see the sickness on their face, they were pale and gaunt and sad.

But they couldn't stop. The urge to punish themself was too strong and it wouldn't leave them alone, it clung to their back and forced them to carry it around everywhere.

The thing with habits meant to punish is that each time we become accustomed to them they become normal and no longer bring us enough discomfort to fit the brief. I know this from my own disordered eating. Every time we set ourselves a goal of restriction, when that amount of food becomes normal it no longer feels like restriction. So we move the goalposts, again and again and again, until we vanish, or until someone intervenes.

In Jules' case, they were the one to intervene, but it was their body rather than their mind that did so. As their energy levels dropped and they started to become dizzy and faint, Jules realized they had a medical problem. They started getting aches and pains all over their body, their legs began to hurt and felt brittle and frail. When it got to a point where they could no longer make it to class or do any of their daily activities, they decided to see a doctor.

Their doctor in Brussels was kind and attentive, and he seemed determined to help them. He ran blood tests and checked their vitals and could tell that something was wrong, but he didn't know what. Going back and forth to the doctors was frustrating and draining, and robbed Jules of the little energy they had left.

Eventually, Jules got a diagnosis: Hashimoto's disease. It is an autoimmune disease that causes the body to attack the thyroid gland until the gland becomes diseased and swollen. It causes tiredness and fatigue. As with so many autoimmune disorders, doctors aren't quite sure what causes it. But as with so many autoimmune disorders, it is likely to be caused by a body under severe distress.

For the first time, Jules told their doctor about their eating disorder. Could that have caused my thyroid to break down? they asked.

Yes, he nodded solemnly.

Hashimoto's is a permanent condition. Again, as with so many autoimmune diseases, there is no known cure. Jules takes medication every day to support their thyroid, and they will probably have to do that for the rest of their life.

．　　　．　　　．

When I speak to Jules and Ingrid and Pat, I feel furious at the world for forcing them to pretend to be less complicated than they are. I feel guilty for all the times – and there have been many – that I have perpetuated the idea of gender as either binary or destiny, when it is neither. I feel enraged when I think about how little effort people make to understand them.

I am so lucky. I have never struggled with my gender identity. I have always felt completely at home as a woman. My first experience of trying to change my body was those obsessive nights munching on chicken wings in the dark in the mid-2000s, trying to grow hips and thighs and breasts. My biggest problem was wanting to either be more or less of what I already was. What a luxury.

That means I will never understand what it's like to be gender-fluid or to struggle with being identified the way I wish to be by others. But I want to try. I think about all the pressure on them to be a false self, and how much strength it takes to throw off that imperative. How much possibility it opens up when you do.

CHAPTER FIVE

I wanted to write something about body image, and I also wanted to write about beauty. But then I realized that in the age of the Instagram influencer the idea of one 'body image' is outdated and archaic. We must now be a thousand body images – a mosaic of constantly updated frozen selves for the grid or the story, all curated but appearing effortless. Our body image is only valid if we can replicate it ad infinitum, if we can get others to show an outward expression of approval. It is about proving every day that we are beautiful, without trying to be beautiful. So it is more than a series of body images; it is a life image. It shows us looking good and thin but also healthy and empowered and smart and well-read and quirky and able to take a joke.

Social media is the ultimate leveller, they say. Anyone can post anything they want. But here's the dark underbelly of that feature: social media has democratized beauty. Ten years ago, when I was a teenager, beauty and thinness were things we saw in glossy magazines but not in our own lives. Celebrities and their beauticians and workout routines were something we loved to follow, but we had a healthy sense that their world was not *our* world. We would, of course, buy the products in the magazine to try and look like them, but we never really expected they would work, and we were okay with that. Picture-perfect beauty standards were reserved for the ultra-rich and famous.

But that's not the case any more. Somewhere along the line, the explosion of Instagram and Snapchat has blurred the lines between our own lives and the ones we read about in print. When Instagram started marketing itself as a platform to follow brands and celebrities plus the people you actually know, something buckled. The two worlds came crashing into one another.

I scroll through photos of models on Instagram all day, every day. Every time I post a photo I spend at least an hour deciding whether I look thin enough and pretty enough. I see all my friends doing it too. If a stranger picked up my phone, they wouldn't be able to tell the difference between my friends and the actresses and models I follow. That is a very big problem.

Every time I open Instagram, I feel sick. I look at the models and compare their photos to mine and feel a crushing sensation in my chest. I expect myself to look and dress like them even though looking and dressing immaculately is their full-time profession. I work full time as a journalist and I write books on the side. Yet I still always find time to curate the perfect Instagram post.

Research has persuasively showed that the advent of Instagram has had a disastrous effect on girls' and women's body image. A 2016 paper, 'A Systematic Review of the Impact of the Use of Social Media Networking Sites on Body Image and Disordered Eating Outcomes', published in the international peer-reviewed journal *Body Image*, found that photo-based activities, like scrolling through Instagram, are destructive to our body image and sense of self. Scholars attribute this to 'social comparison theory' – the idea that having friends and celebrities on the same platform leads us to compare ourselves equally to both categories.

A 2019 study, 'Social Media and Body Image', by Project Know, a charity designed to help people with addictive behaviours, showed that social media can exacerbate eating disorders and trigger certain genetic or psychological predispositions to addictive behaviour. While social media hasn't been definitively proven to cause psychological disorders, the study found, it can exacerbate underlying mental health conditions. We seek out comparison like an addiction to any other substance used to numb the feeling of shame.

In a survey of 227 female university students, 'Negative Comparisons About One's Appearance Mediate the Relationship Between Facebook Usage and Body Image Concerns', which was published in the journal *Body Image*, women reported that while browsing Facebook they tend to negatively compare their own appearance with their peer group and with celebrities, but not with family members. The comparison group that had the strongest link to body image concerns was distant peers, or acquaintances.

This rings true to me – there is something about that illusive third category of comparison that Instagram has created: people you have some distant social connections with but are not actually close to. These people and their curated lives easily blur into the celebrity category – but the difference is that we see them at the local pub and pretend we don't Instagram stalk their every move.

Instagram also has a purpose-built reward mechanism: the likes, or even just the promise of them, keeps us coming back for more. I would be willing to bet that likes popping up in push notifications release dopamine in the brain and serve a similar function to the addiction–reward cycle. It certainly does for me. Posting a selfie or a curated life image and watching the likes roll in makes us feel like we have achieved something.

The sense of achievement here is important. It is a nod to the fact that social media saturation has not only transformed beauty into something everyone can and should aspire to, it has also turned it into a moral imperative. The creation of life images has led us to associate polished Instagram pictures with a good, or moral, existence. It's how we show our friends that we are 'doing well', even when – especially when – we are not.

Instagram has become the means by which we convey success and happiness. This takes different forms – professional success, relationship success, self-satisfaction – but no matter what the content, the conduit is always thinness and beauty.

Have you ever scrolled through a best friend's Instagram and felt jealous of her life, even though you know full well it is flawed and imperfect and sometimes desperately sad? Even though you know it is an act? I have.

. . .

I meet Amma over Twitter in 2019. She tells me a story about her body that stretches back into her childhood and ends with a terrible event that happened a few months before we meet. It's amazing to me the way she can put together the story like this, from beginning to end, over the phone to a near perfect stranger one evening in early autumn. She is well-spoken and clever, and I admire her immediately.

Amma pulled herself out of bed on a cold, blustery morning in February and ate three blueberries on the walk between the kitchen and the bathroom on her way to shower.

Before she got into the shower that day, she stared at herself for a long moment through the misty fog. Her eyes were dull and the colour of lager, she thought, and she hated them. She had three pimples clustered between her eyes, in a little triangle, each with a tiny whitehead on top. She stared at her face until the three dots swam into each other, around each other. She squeezed them, hard, with her long nails. She pulled back just before she made herself bleed, because she didn't want to leave a mark, but she found that her thumbs wanted to keep digging, keep pressing, so, as she let her arms fall to her sides, her biceps sore from the strain of squeezing the pimples over and over, she dug her thumbnail into the back of her left ring finger until it bled.

Her fringe flopped over her eyes, heavy with the humidity from the running shower, and it made her look like a goat, she thought. She pulled it back, pinned it, and splashed her face with water. She peeled off her pyjama top, which was thinning and covered in stains and which she loved dearly, and threw it onto the floor. As she stepped out of her trackpants and pulled down her underwear, she was thinking about a poem she had read a few days before. It was called something like 'For the Woman at the United Airlines Check-In Desk', and it had a line in it about all the bodies in Departures, how they were all naked under their clothes, and for some reason the cadence of that line had stuck with her and was playing on a loop in her head now as she bundled her underwear into her trackpants to wash while everyone was out. She stepped under the shower and let it scald her.

She pulled on three pairs of tights underneath her school skirt, because it was freezing and because they made her feel contained. She walked to the bus stop slowly, distractedly, because for some reason she was still thinking about the poem, still trying to remember the line that came after the one about bodies in the departure lounge. She was also thinking about the night before, when she had come across the poem online. She had been scrolling through her Tumblr dashboard, which was something she always did when she was sad, because it was the only social media account she had that was totally private and totally dedicated to writing.

Amma felt she could never tell anyone she was a writer, or even a reader, because her friends at school would tease her viciously. But the truth was that she loved to write, she did it all the time. She loved to mimic her favourite authors and poets, writing verses in her head as she fell asleep, jolting upright when she landed on something good so she could write it down in the notes section of her phone before it disappeared into the night.

Tumblr is full of writers who can't tell anyone they are writers, so she felt at home there. People are known only by their blog name, and Amma could be totally anonymous. She shared poems and passages she loved and she had carefully curated a perfect feed where other writers' work popped up every minute or so and she could get lost in a sentence from Sylvia Plath. The night before, she had been scrolling through Tumblr for hours by the time she came across the airport poem, slowly trying to calm herself after a panicked day. When she found the poem, there was something about its rhythm that settled her. So she had repeated it, those lines about the bodies in the departure lounge, as she fell asleep, and she found herself repeating it again now as she walked.

Amma pulled herself onto the bus heavily when it arrived. The air was icy and the streets were empty; the bus appeared like a spectre trundling down the main road in her town. An hour later, these streets would be full of schoolkids, full of girls her age getting their buses to school. But Amma's grammar school was in a different city, which was miles and miles away from where she lived, and her commute started every morning at 7 a.m. This frozen, quiet hour. The witching hour, she called it. She hated living so far away from school, the one her parents sent her to because she got a scholarship and they said it was too good to turn down. She hated the early mornings, and she hated the green-grey circles they left under her eyes, but she liked the witching hour, because she was always alone in it.

It was half eight by the time she arrived at school that morning, and she was bleary-eyed from sleeping on the bus. As she walked up to the school gates, she was playing her favourite AFI album loudly to calm herself. Her headphones were big and black and expensive and new, given to her by her parents as a present for starting year seven at nearly twelve, a few months earlier. She shuffled into English class, her first lesson of the day, with her headphones still on and the music still playing loudly. The girls next to her sniggered as the thick guitar sound bled into the room. She yanked the cable from her iPod to silence it.

At break time she remembered the pimples between her eyes, because the skin was stinging where she had almost pierced it, and she went to the bathroom to try again to purge them from her face. As she steadied herself in front of the mirror, she realized that the thick black eyeliner she applied on the bus had smudged, so she wiped away the dusty shadow under her eye, pulled the pencil from her bag and reapplied it.

She moved through the day dreamily. Her maths teacher looked disappointed as he handed her back her paper, the first exam of the school year, which she had failed. She hated maths, but the sting of the failure still electrified her, sent goosebumps down her spine. The girls sitting on her table spotted her mark and gave each other sideways looks. Amma wondered why she couldn't go to a school like the ones she saw in American films, where it's cool to be bad at things, to not care, to wear black clothes and black eyeliner and have one headphone on your ear at all times. But no, this was a grammar school in Lancaster, and she would never be accepted or admired here.

She hadn't made a single friend at the school yet, but this didn't surprise her much. She had never found it easy to get along with girls, she had always preferred the company of boys. Here, there were only girls, and they were pretty and rich and wanted nothing to do with her.

After school, headphones still on, she moved towards the door that opened into the playground and was distracted when she reached the door handle. She pulled on it and it swung towards her, but she had underestimated its weight – it was an unusually heavy door – and it didn't swing open quite far enough for her to walk through. She became awkwardly wedged in the half-open door as she tried to leave, the clips on the straps of her backpack making clattering noises as they knocked against the hard wooden doorknobs. Using the back of her right foot, she pushed the door again so there was enough room for her to walk through, but someone had seen her in this moment of unseemly struggle.

A girl called Glenn, like the actress, laughed and said something about the fact that Amma would have an easier time fitting through doorways if she dropped a stone, something about a 5:2 diet, how her mum lost ten pounds in a week, how she would send her a Facebook message later that night with the link. She was smiling and laughing as she spoke and her teeth looked menacing even though they were beautiful, even though she was beautiful.

The girls around her joined in and the laughter became louder, like a siren ringing in Amma's ears. One of them said something about self-control, about how Amma shouldn't eat so many carbs. One of them asked a question, something about how she should join their netball team, which she didn't mean, of course, and even if she had, Amma would rather die than play netball with girls like them.

Her vision blurred slightly as the laughter continued but became muted, as if further away, and Amma started to feel light-headed. She felt as though the steps in front of her were disintegrating, shattering in slow motion beneath her feet, as though the door frame behind her was collapsing, as though every solid structure around her had lost its edges. She held her breath and waited for the feeling to pass. In a few moments, it began to fade, and as her eyes refocused she could see that the girls were walking away, absorbed in a different conversation now, and she was free to go.

Amma stared down at her knees, nestled under three pairs of tights, as she sat on the bus. The windows were icy. She had always, always been teased, she thought, ever since she could remember, for being fat. Not fat, that's not right, but pudgy. Squishy. Soft. The girls at school had taken it to a new level with their constant taunts and their lip gloss and their impossibly thin thirteen-year-old bodies that were somehow still prepubescent even though Amma already looked like a woman.

Amma was familiar with this kind of teasing. But somehow that didn't make it any easier. All the novels she read seemed to say that there are so many things in life that are supposed to get better with time. That you just get used to things, even bad things, even terrible things, and after a while they become bearable. But this had never been true for Amma, not with the taunts.

Amma comes from a fat family, she tells me that night in August when we first speak. That's what she's always thought, she says. She feels as though that phrase means something more than the two words it places together. No one in her family is hugely overweight, no one is stop-and-stare-in-the-fridge-aisle-at-Tesco's fat. No one is unwell. But everyone in the family is on the heavy side, and always has been, and always will be.

Amma tells me that a 'fat family' is constant talk of diets and exercise regimes but no one losing any real weight. It is snide jokes at the dinner table about siblings' puppy fat, and later, when Amma starts wearing tight jeans, it is jibes about muffin tops while watching the football with her brother. It is knowing her brother hates being heavy, hates being loose and flabby but would never admit it, so he plays rugby obsessively until his extra weight becomes something he can crush opponents with. A fat family is a shared slow metabolism and exhaustion with all the ways the different members try to outsmart it. It is being a size 12–14 at thirteen years old, which is fairly normal, but everyone is so used to making jokes about each other's size that Amma gets called pudgy almost every night.

And so Amma always considered herself overweight. She always wanted to be a stone or two lighter, ever since she learned how to weigh herself. On the cusp of year eight, aged twelve, she was impossibly good at wanting to be different than she was.

She constantly feels heavy these days, she tells me. Not just in the sense that she is overweight, although she is, but in the sense that she feels weighed down, like her thighs are full of concrete, like she is trying to walk underwater, like every step she takes is a boulder being dragged along a dirt path.

She hated that the girls at school teased her, but she knew they were right. She was unsightly. As she got older, she saw it more and more and more. She woke up every morning and said *You are disgusting* to herself in the mirror, and the truth was that this was the most hurtful voice of all.

She had started putting on even more weight recently, she tells me, her thighs expanding and her breasts getting heavier, embarrassing her everywhere she went, making her wish she was invisible. She desperately wanted to stop getting bigger.

Since she started high school in the other city Amma had been shaving her legs because she couldn't stand the way the other girls had teased her last September when they noticed the wild hair she let grow there. This time, though, she didn't shave her legs; instead, she reached for her razor and popped the blade out of its casing, just like she had seen girls do on Instagram, and she pushed it into the skin at the top of her leg. She pulled the blade out again and inspected her work, saw that she had created a one-inch-long crater. She pulled the skin apart and saw ash-white flesh for a moment, before it started to fill with blood. She watched the bright red blood collect, and she quietly congratulated herself on this poetic synchronicity. It had now been two months since this discovery, and each time her legs got bigger she sliced into them, and now there was a little cluster of vertical cuts lined up next to each other, neat and straight like a tally, like she was keeping count of something.

As she grazed her hand across her thighs on the bus, feeling the bumpy skin beneath her tights, she thought about a blackboard she used to have above her bedhead in primary school. She had asked her parents for it with dreams of becoming an artist, a chalk-master, learning to create drawings that would one day hang in museums. Instead, the blackboard was mostly blank and unused, except for one week every year around Christmastime. Her best friend, Joe, went away to see his dad's family in Ireland every year between Christmas Eve and New Year. Amma hated her home city without him, couldn't stand it, it felt so dull and cold and grey and suffocatingly vast. She always dreaded the week he wasn't there, because her loneliness closed in on her so quickly the moment he was gone.

So every year on the day he left, he would come to her house and they would listen to AC/DC on iTunes and talk about New Year's resolutions until his father came to collect him, saying it was time to go to the airport. When their car pulled out of Amma's driveway, Dublin-bound, crunching through the snow, she would pick up a piece of yellow chalk and draw a line on the board, representing the first day he was gone. Each night when she went to bed, she would add one mark to the tally and would feel grateful that she had survived one more day without him. On the fifth day, she would draw the yellow chalk across the four lines to make a bundle, and this always satisfied her. As she thumbed the cuts in her legs she thought of those tallies, how the lines in chalk were a bit like the lines she'd drawn across her legs, and she briefly wondered what it would feel like to draw them together like she did with every fifth chalk mark, dragging a blade diagonally through a line of still-healing wounds.

.   .   .

When I speak to Amma about high school, a clear memory swims back to me. I remember standing in line at a theme park on a much-anticipated end-of-year school trip, holding both my arms across my body to cover it and the bikini I can't remember why I chose, pretending to be cold and shivering so I had an excuse to curl my arms around myself like a fortress. I spent weeks deciding what to wear, because we didn't have to wear uniforms for the day and I knew the boy I liked would sit near me on the bus. He was in a different class to me, so we rarely got to spend this kind of incidental time together – the kind of time where knees brush against knees and you can pretend there is nothing you can do about it, where you can think carefully about every little movement, let him catch you in what he thinks are candid moments, staring into space, where he might think to himself, *Wow, she looks just like the dream girls in the movies.*

He didn't sit next to me on the bus, but it was OK because I just played Snake II on my phone and pretended I wasn't interested in talking to anyone.

The day passed in a blur, with so much excitement that my stomach felt as though it had been emptied out. I promised myself I would not go swimming all day – it was a water theme park – because I needed to make sure no one saw me in my bikini. But it was the end of the day and one of the teachers had accused me of being a 'bad sport', and the only thing I hated more than myself was displeasing other people, so I gritted my teeth and approached the water slide.

This is how I ended up in the line, clutching myself, digging my fingernails into the skin on my arms. There was giggling behind me, a bunch of boys and a few girls, and I turned to see the boy I liked standing behind me, saying, Don't turn around, Lucia, you're only hot from behind. I was about to turn thirteen.

There are photos of this day, grainy, pixelated, taken by the one girl in our year who had a camera phone in 2004. A Motorola. The photos of us smiling next to water slides got texted between us via MMS message the day after the excursion. I remember the photos so clearly because it was one of the first times friends and I were able to share photos of ourselves without a disposable camera, or without permission to take our parents' digital cameras out of the house. Something stirred inside me when I saw the picture message on a friend's phone – I couldn't receive MMSs on my Nokia. I was so nervous because I remembered that someone had taken a photo outside the water slide, of us all standing together and smiling just moments before it was my turn to go on the ride. The phone got passed around, and there it was, and my stomach flipped and then settled. I had managed to completely cover myself up in the photo, and I could have kissed the tiny flip-phone screen.

This was the first time I felt the buzz. What an achievement. I had got away with something impossible. There was nowhere to post these photos, so I didn't know the full extent of that buzz yet.

It was three years before Mark Zuckerberg would sit down in his dusty college dorm room, having just been dumped, eager to get back at the girl he had lost in the best way he knew how: not by hating her, but by making her hate herself. The most potent poison, he knew. So he coded a program that would compare the faces of two girls in their college to let men – no, boys – vote on which of the two was hotter. He would force his ex to suffer under the weight of comparison with this new website he had created.

The first time I hurt myself, I was twelve years old. I was a hyper-competitive young athlete, a gymnast, and my body was the most important thing in the world to me. I was training for my first ever world championships, which would take place in France in 2004. I had been training my whole life for this.

As that year wore on and the big competition started feeling closer and closer, I started getting worried about putting on weight. My best friend from the gym and I used to worry so much at this age because we could see girls around us hitting puberty, getting hips and thighs, and that was the last thing we wanted. Every time we had a sleepover, we promised each other that we would never let ourselves get heavier than thirty-five kilos. We were both around thirty-three kilos at the time; we weighed ourselves every day at home and in a big competition year we had 'weigh-ins' every week at the gym.

(I realize, writing this now, that this would have been the same time I was lusting after a more curvaceous body. What cognitive dissonance, wanting to create and destroy myself at the same time.)

The more I thought about it, the more afraid I was that my body would start changing without my permission. One of my mentors at the gym, a man I admired greatly, used to warn me about puberty, used to tell me it could ruin my career if I let it. He always used to say he needed me to 'stay little'.

One night, after a particularly rough training session, I was in the shower washing the sweat out of my hair and massaging a bruised knee I had fallen onto earlier that evening. I used to have a ritual every night, in the shower, where I would put my hands around my thigh and join my middle fingers together on one side and my thumbs together on the other. Then I would slide the completed circle up my leg until I got to the point where I couldn't go up further without my fingers losing touch with one another. It was a test to make sure I *stayed little*.

But this night, I realized that all the skin on my thigh looked the same, so I wouldn't necessarily know if the threshold where I could fit my thigh into my hand was moving slowly down my leg as I got bigger. I needed a permanent way to mark that threshold, so I would always know if I was failing at my own test. I took my father's razor from the shelf in the shower and pulled it clean across my thigh where my hands had been. I still have that scar. Its permanency worked.

.　　　.　　　.

By the time school started that September, Amma still didn't have any friends there, and the bullying had become much, much more vicious. She spent the summer loafing around her home town with Joe and she was happy, but every day she had a moment of dread when she realized that she would soon have to start dragging herself out of bed at 6 a.m. and haul herself to school.

Over the summer the girls had started creating Facebook events for the diet company 'Jenny Craig and the Biggest Loser' and sending her invitations as a joke, which would have been bad enough, except that her parents had left her alone with a new live-in babysitter all summer and she hadn't even eaten a proper meal since the end of May because she was trying hard to be restrained, and she had put on at least half a stone, she guessed, based on the lines etched on her thighs in blood.

Amma's parents are working class, both nurses for the NHS, and they struggle to keep their family together, to make ends meet on their measly salaries. They were overworked and underpaid, and they had both taken on second jobs that year. They were pulling day and night shifts at the local hospital and were hardly ever at home, so they brought all sorts of people into the house to watch the children.

Amma was thirteen, so she really should just have been left alone, but her parents insisted. They knew she was lonely at school, and that she and her brother had stopped getting along lately, so Amma suspects they just wanted an excuse to force someone to keep her company. The people they got were great – really eclectic, usually travelling through the city on some big adventure, people who needed a place to sleep and crash in the spare room and didn't need to be paid very much. Amma really liked them. They are, she thinks, some of the only people she met that year that she actually got along with. She sensed that they were outsiders too, and she liked hearing their stories. They were never anything like the girls at school.

But the downside of this was that invariably these ragtag friend-babysitters were hopeless in the kitchen, and they made pasta every night, even when Amma tried to get them to let her cook, so she had been putting on weight all summer, and she was terrified about what the girls at school would say.

It was windy but warm, the kind of autumn day Amma likes, when school went back. She was turning fourteen next month, which meant she could start applying for jobs at the high street record stores, and the thought of creating a life that looked like the movie *High Fidelity* buoyed her through the day.

She had been moved down to a lower maths class, she discovered in first period, which was not surprising but gutting all the same. When she walked into biology the gaggle of girls in her old maths class were sitting there and they immediately asked her why she hadn't been in class that morning. Their eyes were twinkling because they knew the answer.

I got dropped to Mr Matthews' class, she whispered, and they feigned sympathy. She moved to walk away, but one of the girls stopped her.

How was your summer? she asked.

Amma stumbled over her answer, trying to say something cool about Jude, the man staying in her spare room, but it came out sounding desperate. What about you? she asked the girl who spoke to her.

Can't complain! the girl chirped. She started telling a story about a new personal trainer she had found on Instagram. Amma had managed to avoid Instagram so far, but she could tell that her absence from the app was exacerbating her social isolation.

Amma had let herself get so carried away with the conversation that she had forgotten her usual routine of scoping out a good spot to sit, near the back, so she could read her book under the desk without being noticed. She looked around and realized the classroom was almost full. The only seat free was the one she was now standing in front of, which people must have assumed she planned to sit in, although she absolutely did not. It was right next to the Instagram girl, who now had her phone out and was looking expectantly at Amma. Amma shuffled into the seat, her mind racing, her vision blurring slightly, looking for a line of a poem to repeat in her head until she could focus again.

. . .

Susie Orbach wrote the seminal anti-diet book *Fat Is A Feminist Issue* in 1978. In her follow-up book, *Bodies*, in 2009, she says things have regressed. Despite all the progress women and girls have made in the last few decades, our body anxiety has worsened. How can that be?

Orbach writes:

> A constant fretfulness and vigilance take hold for many from the moment they wake until the time they fall asleep. Their bodies are on high alert. The norm has become to worry. In another time, we would have called such anxieties an illness and, given how many suffer, we would have called it an epidemic. But we don't.

The moralizing of the body and the democratizing of the internet coincide in a very important way: they create ultimate individual accountability for the self and the brand, and the body and face are how we judge the worthiness of that self. The body, Orbach writes, has become a worthy personal project.

When packaged like this, I think I am starting to understand how it is that I justify being a feminist as well as being someone who spends hours each day editing selfies. My individual power has become linked to my image more than ever – if my Instagram posts are shiny and perfect, more people will read my writing about rape. So the calculation becomes a kind of utilitarian one: I can justify participating in an ideological framework with which I disagree in order to get my message to as many people as possible. But how is the message itself not fatally diluted by this process?

In her essay collection *Trick Mirror*, Jia Tolentino writes about how the internet has turned our lives into an endless performance, with aesthetic perfection the ultimate goal because of how strongly we have equated it with moral value or professional success.

In physical spaces, Tolentino writes, 'there's a limited audience and time span for every performance. Online, your audience can hypothetically keep expanding forever, and the performance never has to end.'

Instagram likes are infinite. You can keep piling them up forever, feeling slightly calmer with each one, tricking yourself into thinking there is an amount of social approbation that will quell the very anxiety it has created. There isn't.

In 1959, the sociologist Erving Goffman laid out a theory of identity that revolved around 'playacting'. In every human interaction, he wrote in *The Presentation of Self in Everyday Life*, a person must put on a sort of performance, create an impression for an audience. But the key to the social theory is that there is always a backstage – where you and the other players can cast off the masks and be yourselves with each other – after the final curtain call.

But, as Tolentino notes, on Instagram there is no backstage. The mask must be so convincing that it must look like real life, which means you can never take it off. Have you ever asked a friend to take down a photo of you where you don't look perfect, lest the audience catch you unawares? I have.

Neuroscientist Norman Doidge explains in *The Brain's Way of Healing* that in the term 'body image', the second word is doing a lot more work than we think it is. We think of body image as being the way we appraise our physical body – and therefore that the primary source is the physical body itself. Not so, I'm afraid.

Doidge writes that the body image is formed in the mind and is represented in the brain, then is unconsciously projected onto the body. Neuroscientists sometimes call this the 'virtual body' to emphasize that it has an existence in the brain and mind that is independent of the actual corporeal body. The body image – our sense of our physical body – is a creation of the brain. The physical body is one input that creates this image, but it is far from the only, or the most important, one.

The body image, Doidge says, is built up with input from multiple brain maps, including vision but also touch, pain and proprioception, even the parts of our brain that map sensory or even emotional information about our bodies. Sometimes our brain's map of our bodies matches up with our physical selves. But sometimes it does not. Sometimes it is more heavily determined by our sense of touch – for example, the effect my rape had on my body – than by our sense of sight. Sometimes it is informed by feelings of shame and worthlessness that are neurologically attached to the body – because of something that has happened to it, or something that has been said about it – but which have little, if anything, to do with the properties of the physical body. The brain can cause confusion about which image of our bodies is real and which one is not.

It's no wonder, then, that the advent of platforms like Instagram has wreaked havoc on the brain's map of the body. We have managed to roll multiple significant emotional and moral value judgements into one place, where the focus is ultimately on a visual representation of the body or face.

This gets me thinking about perfectionism. Mine, and others'. I think there is some equivalence between obsession about thinness and beauty and obsession with achievement more generally. I think – at least in my case – that my perfectionism comes from a desperate attempt to prove that I am worth something. To fight the little voice in my head that says over and over: *You are a filthy rotten thing.* If I can find as many external markers of success as possible, something I can point to and say look, this is who I am, then I am granted some reprieve from the voice's death-grip. I become obsessed with outrunning myself, outperforming myself, in ways that other people can witness. Instagram likes serve exactly the same purpose.

Perfectionism is also closely related to shame. Psychiatrist Robert Karen says in his paper 'Shame', published in *The Atlantic Monthly*, that adults who grow up feeling a strong sense of shame in themselves often seek an addictive or compulsively busy lifestyle so that unwanted self-images can be kept hidden. Imagine, then, the impact of a combination of shame, perfectionism and an endlessly regenerative platform to illustrate success. Perhaps the seventy-two minutes we spend on average every week taking selfies is just another form of numbing, another kind of overachievement.

.   .   .

It was a Friday in June, years later, and Amma had planned a trip back to her home city for the weekend to visit her friends. Joe and Michael and Trey had organized a dinner party in her honour, and she was excited to see them. They were the only thing she missed about home.

They sat at the dinner table and talked about university and jobs and rental prices and Brexit. She and Joe still talked on the phone every day, even though she lived far away, so she still knew every detail of his life intimately. But the others she had lost touch with, so she sat back and listened to their updates, their Tinder war stories, their tales of drunken nights out at the club they all used to sneak into when they were seventeen.

After dinner, they decided to go to a house party down the road from the boys' house. It was sticky and smelled like beer. Amma drank vodka and tonic all night and told the boys about the bookshop where she worked, and she felt something like pride.

She and Joe left the party to have a cigarette outside – something Amma never normally did, but she was drunk and feeling reckless, and she liked the way it gave her an excuse to talk to her best friend alone. They walked slowly down the alleyway beside the house, looking for a milk crate to perch on. Joe was swaying slightly; she could tell he was drunk too. He was telling her about his recent break-up, how his ex was crazy and possessive. Amma prickled at this, and wondered whether she should tell him what she thought of this kind of gendered language. While she was considering doing so, she missed her chance, and he had moved on to telling her about someone he had met on a dating app the night before.

She smiled encouragingly and looked at the girl's profile, coo-ing and mmm-ing at her witty bio, complimenting her dress sense.

She's really sexy, Joe said, still slurring, and all of a sudden Amma felt as though there was a bird trapped in her chest. He looked up at her intently, and then he was kissing her, and she didn't know what happened next, but somehow he was holding her throat and he had his fingers inside her. His breath was thick with whisky and beer and stale cigarette smoke and his eyes looked as though they were possessed. She didn't move; she could feel the strength of his arm pinning her down and knew there was no point in trying. She closed her eyes and came to half an hour later, crumpled on the alleyway floor, underwear around her ankles, skirt back to front, bleeding and alone.

. . .

When Amma tells me this story, the rape is six months old. She tells me she used to be a hugger, but she can't touch anyone any more. She won't even hug her parents, she says. Her body feels different. Stiffer. It hurts her sometimes when she lies in bed.

She asks me if this feeling ever goes away.

I read your book, she says, after she sees that I am taken aback by her comment.

She is talking about *I Choose Elena*. I pause for a long moment as I wonder about the ethics of this. Can I answer her question? Or must I stick to asking them? As a journalist, is it okay for me to speak about this thread that connects us? It is, after all, I am starting to realize, probably why she reached out to me in the first place, when

I asked my Twitter following if anyone was interested in speaking to me for this book.

By offering up my own story, have I forever compromised my ability to see hers clearly? Can I move between subject and narrator in this way without undermining the project? Can I tell Amma's story now that I know how connected it is with my own?

The answer to her question, I think, is no, not really. There are some things you never get back. I don't say this. Maybe I should have. Instead, I say nothing.

I think of a poem I love by Blythe Baird, which ends with the lines:

A few hours before my best friend raped me on our college campus,
We discussed the prospect of astro-projection.
He couldn't understand why I wanted to experience it so badly.
Why would anyone want to leave their body, he laughed.
And in this moment,
We have nothing
In the world
In common.

CHAPTER SIX

When I meet Farhana at a cafe in central London in 2019, she is twenty. She is confident and self-aware. She knows more about her body, it seems, than I do even now at twenty-seven. I think about how lost I was at her age, how lost I still am.

Farhana has always chased boys who don't like her back. Or at least, the ones who won't admit to liking her back. This boy was probably the same, but she couldn't stop thinking about him.

She was sitting in her university seminar one day – she studies geography – when she realized he was flirting with one of the other girls as well as her. They walked in arm in arm, and the boy was smiling from ear to ear. He looked so pleased with himself, she tells me. The girl he had chosen was one who had always been particularly cruel to Farhana. She had made snide comments about Farhana's skin, her mixed-race, half-Ghanaian, half-British skin, microaggressions that wore on Farhana day after day, ones that this friend would probably accuse her of imagining if she had ever asked her to stop.

She had been on one almost-date with the boy, the week before. He had asked her after class if she wanted to spend the afternoon together, and she had said yes. They'd had a really nice time, walking down the high street, chatting, stopping for hot chips and pizza. Some of the other girls had seen them – including the one he was interlocked with in class – and she could see their jealousy. They were mean, and she knew this moment would come back to haunt her.

In class the next day, she tried not to look at him. He hadn't spoken to her in a week, since their afternoon date. He had ignored her every day at uni since. He had even ignored the two texts she sent him where she'd pretended to be fine with his silence and that she was just 'seeing how he was', but she also knew that her desperation probably showed. Both messages had two blue ticks underneath them, that horrible indicator that he had read them and ignored them.

We are sitting in a restaurant in Angel when she tells me this story. I will never forget the way she describes how his face changed when he saw her that day in class.

It's like he knew he was supposed to feel guilty, but he also didn't really care, she says.

Ha, I think. I have seen that expression on men's faces so many times. That feeling like they know, on some level, that they've mistreated you. That they shouldn't have ghosted you. That they could have taken five minutes to send one text message to explain why they didn't want to continue the relationship. They know they *should* feel bad about this, but they don't. It's a very specific look that I've seen in men's eyes so many times: when they clock you and think, oh god, I should be ashamed, I should feel bad or feel like I need to apologize, but somehow, written on the same face, is the fact that none of this really bothers them at all. That's why the apology never comes. They know they should do it, but they just never get round to it.

It's like he knew he was supposed to feel guilty, but he also didn't really care. Farhana's words have stayed with me for months.

Back in the draughty university classroom, Farhana avoided the boy's eyes like they would turn her to stone. She didn't want to see that look in his face ever again. She didn't want or need his pretend pity. She ignored him, but it didn't work, because he decided to ignore her first.

In Waterloo, she laughs as she tells me this. Sorry, this is so high school.

No, I think. Never apologize. I could listen to her forever.

The boy was still flirting with the girl he walked in with. Tears welled up in Farhana's eyes, and she wished they wouldn't. She hated this. She felt trapped all of a sudden, like there were falcons flapping their great, heavy wings in her chest, trying to get away. She looked around the room for a way out, before reminding herself that she was free to leave whenever she liked. But she really should stay and see this thing through, she thought. She could handle a bit more rejection.

The boy and girl flirted all afternoon, sitting on the floor against the far wall of the classroom. At one point the girl put her legs across the boy's.

Farhana ends her story there during our first interview, and it is several weeks before I see her again. This time when we speak, it has been a month since Farhana and the boy had sex. Or tried to. They had been flirting in class for *months*, that kind of scintillating build-up you only get with the particularly emotionally unavailable boys. They had been talking every day on Snapchat, flirting, so much banter, sending nudes.

Eventually – finally – they left a party together. They barely spoke all night, he was talking to other girls, but she caught him looking over at her several times. So when he did finally come over to talk to her, she was ready with her best intense eyes and slightly aloof tones.

When they got back to her home in Romford, she sneaked him up to her loft room without her mother noticing. He kissed her hard and she liked it, but something caught in her throat. She ignored it. Farhana had had sex plenty of times before. It had never been comfortable for her but it had never been a problem, either. She knew what to do.

·   ·   ·

Listening to Farhana's story makes me think about the connection between sex and attachment. About emotionally unavailable people who draw us in somehow, who suck out all of our energy but are somehow still empty.

I never questioned the fact that I hated sex – truly hated it – because I always believed it was a conduit for the closeness I craved.

When I first went to see a sex therapist, I assumed our work would be all about physical pleasure. But I quickly realized that I couldn't resolve the suffering of my body without addressing the relationships I had forced it to give me access to.

I have never once been able to enjoy sex. Even that is an over-statement – I have barely been able to even tolerate it. Every sexual experience I have ever had has been a combination of distinct horrors.

Physical closeness makes me feel as though I am about to jump out of my skin. I loathe it. It fills my throat with angry bees and turns my stomach. Kissing is sometimes enjoyable, as long as it does not feel overtly sexual.

Being naked in front of a romantic partner makes me want to die. I can't stand the sight of myself, the smell. I can't stand the truth of my body, not even for a minute.

Whenever another person touches me, I think about how it feels like they are touching the skin on my elbow. There is almost no feeling at all. No sensation. No arousal. Just nothing.

Over years and years of engaging with sexual partners, I never even considered this. Isn't that funny? Something that I had always been taught was supposed to be pleasurable was completely meaningless to me, and for some reason I never thought to investigate this fact. I think it's because I was keeping my rape a secret, and when I had thoughts about my sexual dysfunction I couldn't help but connect the two, and I didn't want to connect the rape to anything, didn't want it to exist at all, so I pushed the thoughts away and got on with it.

If a man tried to put a finger inside me it felt like my insides were being hacked at with a knife, the pain was so acute. But I pushed through it, because I thought this is what I had to do in order to be worthy of love.

Penetrative sex was almost unbearable. One surgeon used to ask me whether the pain was worse on insertion or deep penetration, and I honestly couldn't answer him. Every moment felt like torture. After a few moments of sex, though, I would dissociate completely.

I would leave my body behind, leave it alone in the torment I had walked it into. I would have the sensation that I was floating above myself, watching, thinking: *Whore.*

It was only years later, after I had disclosed the rape, that my psychoanalyst told me that there are specialist therapists who can help the body recover and become sexually functional. I had never even considered this possibility. I had resigned myself to the idea that sex would be a necessary evil for me, something I had to endure, like vegetables or exercise, to be happy and healthy.

But my first sex therapist, in Sydney, said to me on my first appointment: I want you to promise me you will never again think of sex as something you have to tolerate. I made her that promise, and I kept it.

With Tanya, we mostly worked on physical sensations. She asked me to describe my experience of sex to her and I was honest about it for the first time in my life. When I had finished describing how painful it is, she asked: So why do you do it?

Because it's the only way I can get people to stay, I said.

When I think about this answer now, it breaks my heart. It betrays three things I have now learned a lot about in therapy. The first is that I have always, either because of my rape or the persistent rape culture I live in, connected sex with worthiness and thought that my appeal to the opposite sex was a useful objective signifier that I am not as disgusting as I think I am. The second is that seeking validation from the very thing that makes me feel unworthy in the first place is a form of self-harm. The third is that I am abjectly afraid of abandonment.

As I speak to Farhana over dinner in Angel about her body, I keep thinking about how her intelligent observations could also apply to something that had happened to me earlier that year. I was in a club somewhere in London, lost in my own thoughts as I danced.

Hello, said a voice beside me that I did not recognize.

I swerved around to face it, unsure why my reorientation had been so dramatic, keenly aware that my overreaction had alarmed him.

Oh, sorry, he said. Did I scare you?

No, I said, of course not. Sorry.

As my mind focused more sharply on the man in front of me, I began to take him in. He was tall, and fit, and had what struck me as a particularly kind smile. But his eyes were unfocused. He was drunk and looked like a puppy that had grown slightly dizzy from a game of fetch. I felt mildly uneasy around drunk men, but I had always found a way to quell the feeling. I had had a great deal of practice. So I silenced the faint quiver in my heart and told myself to give him a chance.

At that moment, the S Club 7 song playing over the speakers next to my head ended and transitioned into Michael Jackson's 'Thriller'. The dance floor roared with approval, and I felt – just for a moment – dizzy again. I had watched *Leaving Neverland* for work that week and my head was full of the voices of Jackson's victims describing his sexual abuse to camera. The documentary had thrown me, and I had started having dreams about it, and I couldn't understand why it wouldn't have had this same effect on others. The group of boys I had come to the club with had all watched it, I knew that, because they'd had a debate about it over dinner the week before, but they were happily moving to the tune and performing the obligatory hand movements. This puzzled me, and it made me feel far away from them.

I turned back to the man with the kind smile. He had stopped dancing and was standing still, staring at me. There's no way I'm dancing to this, he said. Want to go get a drink?

I was relieved: I had been right about him. He *is* kind.

I wondered if he had noticed that I, too, had been uncomfortable, and concluded that he hadn't, and that he was just a rare example of someone who cared about this kind of thing even while no one was watching. I hadn't yet learned enough about men who speak so loudly about being on your side that you miss the fact that they are not on your side at all.

The writer Sam Mills has given this phenomenon a name in 'Chauvo-Feminism', her essay about the #Me Too movement. She calls these men 'chauvo-feminists'. According to Mills, the chauvo-feminist is 'the abusive man who hides in plain sight'. He knows that overt misogyny is no longer tolerated, so he hides it, compartmentalizes it. He performs feminism without actually believing in it. He tweets the right articles and says the right things, but when you get him alone, you find out it was all an act.

'His chauvinism is select,' Mills writes, 'targeted at women whom he can manipulate easily, whom he perceives as lacking the power to stand up to him.'

On this night, I was one of those women. I smiled at his offer, accepted it, and followed him to the bar.

I asked if he had seen the documentary about Michael Jackson, and he said yes, and we talked about it for twenty minutes. I was impressed that he had the vocabulary to talk about abuse, and #MeToo, and he seemed to have put some real thought into it. He was smooth, and I was aware of that, and aware that I was so often drawn to people who were good at pretending, but again, I waved away the thoughts and focused on his body language, his eyes, the way his smile got so animated when I told him I was a journalist.

I'm a writer too! he said. Then he told me about his band and his solo music project, about songwriting, about following his dreams. I liked that he identified me as someone who had done the same thing. I felt eminently visible to him in this moment, and the feeling was addictive. So, without thinking, I launched into my routine – tried and true.

That sounds amazing, you must be so talented! It's so great to meet someone who is so dedicated to their work.

I watched the one-liners pour out of me, as I had so many times before, and watched them fill him up like water pouring from a jug into a glass, I watched him stand taller and taller by the minute, watched him settle in to my compliments, watched him ask for more, watched how full he looked when I obliged. The man – whose name, I now know, is Alex – could not believe his luck.

I like being around you, he said, by which he meant *I like the way I feel about myself when I'm around you*. I brushed the thought aside.

I smiled coyly and he leaned in to kiss me, and I was filled with a sense of achievement – no, of relief – that I had held his attention, that he wanted to be physically close to me.

Do you want to get out of here? he asked, smiling that kind smile.

Yes, I said in a voice I did not recognize. It always seems to me that in these moments I become someone else, intoxicated by my own success, totally apart from the rest of my life.

I've only recently come to understand that my dysfunctional attachment styles – my desperate need to please, my conviction that I must be almost invisible if I am to hold on to love, my need to never ask for help – are all about how my body was treated as a child, and as a teenager, and even now, as an adult. That's true for all of us. The body keeps secrets for us that we do not remember.

.　　　.　　　.

Back in Angel, Farhana is telling me what happened next with the boy after they left the party together.

He pulled Farhana's clothes off quickly, he was almost businesslike. She could sense that he didn't want to kiss her as much as she wanted to kiss him, so she stopped.

He held her face for a moment, and she thought he was going to kiss her slowly, like he could tell she wanted it. But he didn't; he held her chin and then grazed her cheek, moving his hand to the side of her face, then to the back of her head and pressed her face downwards, so gently he could almost argue plausible deniability. She complied.

They were standing close together, next to her bed. He had undressed her but they hadn't even reached the bed yet. She got down on one knee, then two. She unbuttoned his jeans and pulled them down, carefully, bringing his underwear with them but being careful not to knock his erect penis as she went. She always worries about this. It's a delicate negotiation, this part.

She was on autopilot. Eventually, he stopped her.

I want to fuck you.

She smiled up at him and stood up, relieved. She walked over to the bed and lay down.

She was drier than usual. She wanted him – she did – but her body was not cooperating. He kissed her now – finally – and moved himself on top of her. But when he tried to push himself inside her, something got in the way. She was not in pain, not really, but he just couldn't get himself inside her. What was happening?

He pushed harder. It was painful now all of a sudden. Very painful. He became a weapon. She pictured a knife trying to pierce tough, scarred skin. Pushing harder, and then breaking through, just the smallest bit, then closing up again. She screamed. He covered her mouth.

When he left, he said he would Snapchat her later. He didn't. He hasn't spoken to her since. Every time she sees him at university, she tells me, she feels sick with rejection and shame. It is an overpowering feeling, she says. Like it might swallow her up. It feels like fear.

She doesn't know what happened that night, but she knows that her body hasn't felt the same since. She knows it scared her. She knows that her eczema, which snakes across her skin when she is anxious and stressed, is covering her arms and legs now, for the first time in years.

When I meet Farhana again, in Shoreditch, it has become so bad that she is wearing her father's baggy t-shirt. Anything else is too painful on her angry skin. She is wearing a black beanie and her hair is dead straight. She tells me she is going to avoid sex for a while. She tells me she is embracing the modesty trend. She says now that she suspects she has vaginismus – a condition she read about in *I Choose Elena*, which she has read since we've started talking. Her doctors agree, she tells me over tacos.

. . .

Vaginismus is a little-known condition that wreaks havoc on women's lives. Sufferers experience an automatic contraction of the vaginal and pelvic floor muscles when any kind of penetration is attempted.

The NHS website says it is an automatic reaction to fear of pene-tration. The sufferer has absolutely no control over how this happens, when it happens, whether it happens. It is an automatic physical reaction, like vomiting when poisoned food hits your stomach. It is not mental, it is physiological. If you don't listen to your body, your body acts for you, it keeps the score.

Women who suffer from vaginismus cannot tolerate sexual penetra-tion, and sometimes penetration of any kind, including using tampons or submitting to vaginal swabs. It can be caused by physical trauma or sexual abuse, but sometimes the causes are not clear.

The writer Daisy Johnson, a professional and personal idol of mine, wrote beautifully about vaginismus for the Wellcome Collection in 2018.

She explains that roughly two in every thousand women suffer from vaginismus. She herself was diagnosed with the condition in 2017. The diagnosis triggered months of appointments, physical therapy, and psychosexual therapy.

She writes:

> I show this essay to a friend and he says: did you know that, etymo-logically, the meaning of 'trauma' is 'wound'? Every woman knows what it is like to laugh about something that isn't funny, to experience harm from the places harm should not come from. These are small wounds, adding up to an enormous rage.

Daisy's doctors concluded that her vaginismus had come from several bouts of pelvic inflammatory disease, an infection of the reproductive organs that causes severe pain. During one of these infections, she was examined by a doctor who used a speculum – a horrible, pene-trative device used to examine the vagina – that was too big for the examination, let alone for a woman suffering from severe pain. He didn't stop when she cried out in pain. These infections and her rough treatment set off an intense fear of pain and, ultimately, vaginismus, her doctors said. Remember what I said earlier in this book about pain taking on a life of its own?

I imagined what I would say to that GP if I saw him, Johnson said. The words were enormous, great balloon animals in my head. I would say: 'This is what it's like to have a vagina. This is what it's like when no one listens when you tell them to stop.'

When we arrived at his house, Alex showed me his guitar collection before grabbing hold of me and pushing me against his bookshelf, kissing me with the force of a thousand unfulfilled nights, fumbling with my shirt in a way that was so urgent it made me feel transcendent.

The next part was a blur. He muttered something about not having a condom because one-night stands weren't really his thing, and I groaned and let him push himself inside me anyway. It hurt, like knives, but it always does, and I held my breath to create distance between myself and the feeling.

I closed my eyes, pretended to moan with pleasure so I could express some of the pain I was feeling. I think of this as a controlled release. Like the way they intentionally light fires in rural Australia to stop unexpected wildfires from blazing.

Is it that good? he asked. Yes, I breathed, putting my face to his ear so I could have a moment to myself.

The pain didn't really register with me, though, it never really does. It is just part of the process, and it is always worth it because I feel whole afterwards, as though I can relax for a bit, knowing I am wanted in this way, protected by this knowledge no matter how much it makes me suffer.

I grew weary because he was drunk and he couldn't come, but I did not let it show. I was on autopilot, making all the right noises, all the right facial expressions, hoping that if I performed my arousal *just so* it would get him excited enough to finish, and then he would fall on top of me, and then slide out of me, and I would be free to fall asleep, filled with that consuming sense of relief, both that it had happened, and that it was over.

That night I dreamed about a plane crash, and I worried I might have screamed in my sleep. I hope he didn't notice – I didn't want to have to admit to him that I am afraid of flying.

When I woke I felt nauseous from the alcohol and prickly from where he had penetrated me and hazy from the feeling of waking up in a strange bed. I looked over at him and noticed that while he was asleep he no longer seemed kind, but hostile somehow, something in the way he was holding his body, something about the audacity of his nudity, the way his legs were spread wide with his hand resting just above his penis, a half-smile on his face as he slept, comfortable and at ease.

He woke up and started kissing me, both aggressively and sleepily. I felt like there were bugs under my skin as he touched me. He tried to push himself inside me again, but my muscles were bound shut. This doesn't happen to me every time I try and have sex, but it is fairly common. I knew straight away that there was no getting around this; my body just wasn't going to let this happen.

I muttered something and climbed over him, collected my earrings from his bedside table, got dressed in the dark, called myself an Uber and ran downstairs. It was 7 a.m.

As I got into the car I felt as though I was exhaling for the first time since I had begun holding my breath the night before, while he was inside me, to create a barrier between his body and mine.

I relaxed into the back seat, feeling a strange sense of safety, which makes no sense as there had been no danger, not really, and I closed my eyes against the window of the car and fell into a peaceful sleep.

I jolted awake as the Uber pulled up in front of my flat and all of a sudden I felt hot with shame. I felt a wave of nausea, but nothing followed it except more heat in my throat. I was thinking about the moment from the night before when Alex had slapped my arse, hard, and said something mildly aggressive. I could tell it was just something he was into, and I get this a lot, so at the time I had pushed it to the back of my mind, but now it was creeping back. There was something about this replay that I could not bear, something much more sinister than it had felt when it was happening. I wanted to stop thinking about it so I squeezed my eyes closed, as if this might shut off the images, but it did not, so I opened them again and rushed inside.

I called my editor to tell him I would be late for work. I cannot say why I did this, but something made me feel certain I needed to be alone for at least a few hours. I climbed into bed and turned off all the lights, but the scene wouldn't stop playing, so I dug my thumbnail into the skin on my wrist until it burned, and then I let go, and as I did, I drifted into sleep.

I woke again around 11 a.m. I put on a work shirt and my glasses and started marching to the Tube, firing off emails to bosses. As I neared Finsbury Park station, my phone pinged. It was Alex.

Hey. I had so much fun last night! Shame you had to rush off early. Again sometime?

I felt guilty all of a sudden. He had been kind. He had had a nice time. He hadn't felt what I had felt, the white-hot shame, the stabbing pain. How was he to know? He seemed so nice. And he disapproved of Michael Jackson, so I was sure he hadn't realized he was hurting me. Plus, it thrilled me that he wanted to see me again, so I replied:

Yes please.

I smiled to myself all the way to work.

A few weeks later, we saw each other again. We had been on three dates since I had met him on the dance floor, all within a few days of each other. Something quiet inside me warned that this was probably unhealthy, dangerous somehow – like I shouldn't trust his puppy-dog interest.

What are you doing tonight? Wanna hang? Alex said.

Yes please, I wrote back, and within a minute we had agreed to meet at the pub on my road. It was freezing as I stepped outside, almost snowing, and I wrapped my scarf three times around my face as I walked towards him. He had the cheekiest smile, and he seemed so innocent to me. He kissed me, and I liked it, and we walked inside. My dates with him had been the first time I had let anyone touch me since, well, that last August, when I had inexplicably stopped being able to bear having my last boyfriend's hands on me in bed. I figured this was progress, then, that my body was happy to let Alex touch it, even though I did not know him from a bar of soap.

We drank too much that night and talked excitedly. He was interested in my work, far more so than my last boyfriend had ever been, and I liked that he could talk to me about it. I knew who I was when he talked.

I almost didn't notice that all the conversations we had about me were, in truth, conversations about how my success reflected back on him.

We drank another bottle of red wine and I giggled when he told me my lips had turned maroon. I caught myself thinking about men who needed an audience, about the gaze I was – again – offering to someone who wanted it far too much.

Mostly, we talked about him, and his budding career as a poet. He had always wanted to be a writer, and he was giving it his best shot, and I liked that about him. I was slightly uncomfortable when he said: I just want people to see who I am as an artist, before I become too much of a big deal, you know? But as was my habit, I brushed away the discomfort and focused on the reflection he saw when he looked at me.

We stumbled back to my flat a few hours later. He smelled like my last boyfriend, like my father, like stale beer and disappointment. But I ignored that, too.

To my great surprise, I found that I was almost excited to have sex with him. I wanted him inside me, near me, I craved his touch instead of being repulsed by it.

He kissed me and undressed me, taking only a few moments to do all this before pushing himself inside me. I was not ready, and just like that first night, the night we had met, it felt as though he was plunging a knife into me. I turned my face away, feigning pleasure again, so I could bite down on my tongue and make sure he didn't see my pain. It worked, and he just pushed into me harder, which is what I had wanted, but the pain was almost intolerable now. I closed my eyes and told myself it would soon be over, and I dug my nails into him to try and offset the pain inside me, and I drifted away, and away, and away.

He did not notice I was not there. He pulled my feet together, above my head, so I could no longer see his face and he could no longer see mine. He was pounding into me now, faster and harder, and I thought I might break.

I was terrified that Alex would notice how much I had hated the sex, but he didn't. That was amazing, baby, he said, and I could tell he meant it. I hated the way he said *baby* like that, but this was nothing compared to how much I hated myself in that moment, and how much I needed to know that he was still there with me.

He rolled over and fell asleep within minutes, and I was delighted to be alone. For a minute or two, I enjoyed the feeling of having the space to myself again, but then something washed over me. It felt as though I was being crushed by a thousand tonnes of lead, and all of a sudden the disgust I felt for myself was overwhelming. I felt repulsion burn in my throat, I thought of the way he had looked at me when he said *baby*, the way he had dug his fingers into my thighs, clocking the scars but not asking about them. I felt, in this moment, the desperate need to run away, to get as far away from him, from his fingers, as I could.

My flat was small and the bathroom was the furthest room away from the bedroom so, without thinking, I moved towards it and started running a bath. I poked my head back into the bedroom to check that the running water hadn't woken him up.

I went back into the bathroom and climbed into the bath, unsure of what I was going to do next. Something stopped me from taking the scissors to my skin, even though I wanted to. I had a scar on my wrist from a cut I had made with my thumbnail in the Uber on the way back from his house a few weeks before, and I had started to become worried about how obvious this new habit of mine was. No, it didn't matter, I just needed this feeling to pass. I needed to not feel this disgusted with myself. I picked up the scissors, and put them down again, and in one swift motion, I pushed my fingers down my throat, scratching my tonsils, until I vomited an ocean of red wine into the bathtub. I kept going, again and again and again until I was dry-retching, the only thing coming up small clumps of bile and blood from where I had scratched the back of my throat. I did this in a frenzy, like I was not in control of my own hands, and when I was finished I felt as though I had woken up from a dream. I looked around me and the bathtub was more vomit than water, the smell was putrid, the clumps of red wine and French fries even more repulsive to me than my own body in that moment. I did not know why I had wanted so badly to get everything out of me, but now that it was here, external to me, I felt as though it had been the right thing to do.

I drained the bath, then filled it again, drained it, filled it, drained it, until I was satisfied that the rancid smell had mostly been washed away. I dried myself with a towel and as I did so I looked at myself in the mirror, and it occurred to me that I had never been so perplexed by anything in my life.

I crawled into bed next to Alex, who was still snoring, and eventually I must have fallen asleep. We woke the next day and he suggested we go for brunch, and I agreed, because I liked that this was a sign of his puppy-dog-like approval of me. He could not get enough. I was back in my element by mid-morning: clean, clear-eyed, witty, sharp. I made jokes about the president and the news cycle and I started to feel calm again. We ordered coffees and were about to order food when the coffees arrived. Alex told the waiter what he wanted to eat, and as he did so, I pulled my flat white to my lips and drank.

My throat burned as though the coffee were made of acid. I had completely forgotten about the night before, about the scratches on my throat and the burning from the bile. I coughed, pretended I had accidentally choked on the coffee, and quickly made an excuse about why I had decided not to order any food.

A few days later, I was telling my sex therapist this story. She asked me why I felt the need to make myself throw up until I was empty, and I honestly couldn't tell her.

I was having such a nice time, I said. I think he really likes me.

She looked puzzled.

Can you see how alarming that is?

I didn't know what she meant.

On the one hand, she said, you are telling me a story about abject suffering. About self-hatred and forced vomiting and wanting to purge, to disappear. On the other hand, you are telling me you had a nice evening. How can those things both be true at the same time? Which one of those recollections is real?

I did not have an answer.

It was like my brain was trying to convince myself that sex was tolerable, but my body knew better. My body felt the need to purge it, to exorcize somehow the shame I felt. My body knew I hadn't felt right about this man since the very first time he touched me, weeks earlier. But my brain kept sending me back, again and again, into the fray.

Farhana says something very similar when we talk about the boy from her university class, who she doesn't speak to at all any more, out of her own choice, not his. She says she thought at the time that he was nice, and kind, and trustworthy. But she also knew he wasn't.

My body knew before my mind did, she says. And I think again about the thing my therapist keeps saying to me, week after week, when I say, I don't know if I like this situation or if I'm afraid of it, I don't know what's real, and she says: But you do. You do know. You are just not listening to the part of yourself that is telling you what you know.

CHAPTER SEVEN

I t seems particularly cruel to me that rape is one of the only crimes you have to simulate, again and again after it happens, for years and years, until you die. This is what angers me so much about rape – it takes something everyday, something that for some is even positive, and turns it into a crime. How do you make sense of that?

So many of the women and non-binary people I spoke to for this book were trying to recover their bodies from rape or sexual abuse. But recovering the body doesn't just mean waiting for it to heal. It means something else entirely: it means reckoning with the fact that you have had to reperform this act again and again, with people you trust, long after the attack. What does that do to intimacy and trust?

Sex after rape always carries shame. So when we feel ashamed with someone new, where do we put it? It is hard not to project it onto that person, the disgust we feel with ourselves. We get confused; we think that it is them who is making us feel disgusted.

And what about when you do finally overcome that barrier, learn to trust, to let go, and despite all you've done to get there, the person lets you down anyway?

I was on my way home with a new boyfriend. We had been to a nice pub and had had a lovely time together. He was tall and very handsome. He was clever and kind. I felt very safe with him. At least, that is what I thought I felt.

If there was one thing I had learned, it was that excavating all the ghosts that haunt you can make them more frightening before it makes them less so. They do not like to be disturbed.

Another thing I had learned was that the brain has a clever way of lying to us about the things we are most afraid of, especially when it needs us to keep going. I cannot tell you how many times I believed I was safe when I didn't really feel it. I think it's a way of making sure we don't give up. If I knew how long the road to safety would be, I never would have started on it.

So that was how I ended up here: in my kitchen, cowering in a corner near the stove. I was naked except for a towel. I was clutching a large glass of wine in my shaking hands. I was afraid.

I had just had sex with my boyfriend. Everything was fine. Everything was *fine*.

We had talked extensively about my complicated relationship with sex and violence for weeks before we slept together for the first time. He was understanding and loving and he was trying so hard. At each juncture, I could tell that he was gentle and exactly the kind of intimate partner I needed.

But then there was a moment. Just one. He complimented me on something I had done, something he liked, and he breathily told me how good it was, and somehow, immediately, I was thrown into a state of distress and self-loathing. I had managed to stay present while we were connected, but as soon as it was over and he made this comment, an image of myself performing this act flooded into my mind and I felt wholly, painfully, wretchedly disgusted with myself. I thought about the power he had over me in those moments. I thought about how vulnerable I was, how exposed. And I couldn't take it. Something in my brain screamed: *Run*.

So that is what I did. The kitchen was the furthest room in the flat from my bedroom. Another thing I had learned that year is that when I am most afraid, I drink. Chardonnay was my numbing agent of choice.

I was gulping down glass after glass on the kitchen floor, waiting for the moment my self-destructive thoughts would become slightly duller, that sweet relief of feeling a little bit less than I actually felt. In that moment I was desperate and I thought about how much I wished I could ingest the alcohol faster. I needed relief now. I needed to go back to my bedroom before my boyfriend noticed that something was wrong. And when I went back, I needed to have reconfigured my cool girl disguise.

It was so hard to accept that I was still so afraid. The truth is that this moment with the new boyfriend plays out in different ways every time I allow a new person to become physically close to me. It is a devastating cycle, made more devastating by the fact that I refuse to see it clearly.

I have done two years of weekly sex therapy and I have written a book about sexual violence and I have allowed that book to be read by all the men and women I have dated since it came out. In this way, I have allowed myself to be seen and I am trying to understand my fear. But there is still an element of it that keeps getting away from me; that keeps plunging me into the traumatic death-grip of revulsion combined with danger. I shame myself for sex and I shame myself for not being better yet.

How is it fair that one person did a bad thing to me over a decade ago and every day since then *I* have been the bad thing? That every step I take away from it is also a step closer to the next thing that will throw me back there, right back where I started, reminding me that one man forced his shame on me when I was a child and now I will forever be ashamed of myself?

It is not just the first rape that makes me afraid. It is every tiny moment of fear – real and imagined – that has crept into my intimate life since then. It is every man who has been too aggressive in the throes of his desire, every man who has guilted me into going down on him when I didn't want to, every man who has forgotten my requests for gentleness in those final moments, every person who can talk about pain but who cannot acknowledge it when it matters most.

It is the fact that every time I convince myself that I am safe, someone reminds me that I am not. I am only ever moments away from a knife and a dark alley; every violation is connected to every other violation. Each one, small or large, serves as a reminder of that slippery slope. Every time I try to overcome my inability to trust, someone proves to me that people cannot be trusted. How do you explain that to someone who is asking you to trust them without it sounding like an accusation? How can you explain that the world you are describing is dangerously real, whether or not they have witnessed it?

I think this is my sharpest gripe with the primacy we assign to romantic love. It forces me, and all of us, to keep exposing ourselves to danger if we are to seek and find it. Always hoping that our instincts, based on our lived experiences, alerting us to danger, are wrong. Always being reminded that they rarely are.

When I told my therapist about cowering in the kitchen after having sex with my new boyfriend, she told me about something called an 'expectational field'. The idea is that if you are taught something fundamental very early on – that you are worthless, that sex is violent – then you will subconsciously seek out people who confirm that belief. When I heard this, it sounded too much like magical thinking to be something I could get on board with. How could these invisible expectational auras mysteriously attract certain kinds of people, again and again? Surely my romantic life is determined mostly by a dating app algorithm, or my morning coffee routine, or the bars I happen to frequent, than by some idea that I am being pulled in certain directions without my knowing?

But she explained that I was misunderstanding the concept, and I was. It's not about the fact of having met someone – that, of course, is random. We all meet thousands of people in our lifetimes. What matters is who we choose to chase, and who we allow to stay. It is about the series of small and big interactions with new people, on the basis of which we decide whether we will pursue them or let them leave. Those moments of ambivalence or nastiness that would make others put the phone down and walk away are the precise moments that pull me in. The questionable moment during sex that would make some people so uncomfortable they would leave is the one that tells me I am home. Better the devil you know.

I slowly began to understand that she might be right. That I really am attracted to people who meet my expectations of romantic intimacy. But this is so cruel, because just like the neuroplastic brain, the repeated patterns cement in our minds that the original foundation – I am worthless – is true. It reverberates again and again. How can you teach your rational mind to reject something your subconscious is hopelessly addicted to?

When I explained to my therapist how anxious and afraid I often felt when I was with my new boyfriend, she said it was interesting that I was forcing myself to continue in a situation that was making me so miserable.

But I have to, I said.

Why? she asked.

Because I have to make it work.

You are forcing yourself to chase something you find unbearable, she says. I have seen you do it so many times.

Do I desperately want this, or do I hate it? Do I need it or not? I feel both of these things as strongly as the other, and I do not know which is real.

I am lying on the grass outside my building during the Covid-19 crisis having a phone conversation with my cousin. I am telling her about a two-day panic I have spiralled into about – another – new boyfriend, and how his texts confirm that he has discovered how toxic and unbearable I am.

They are more distant, I tell her. Definitely.

Are you sure?

Yes.

How do you know?

I can feel it.

I can feel it. And I really can. Does that make it true? Or can the feeling be true without its underlying assumption being based in fact? How is it that my brain can be so easily thrown into chaos by other people?

Doesn't he send you books from Amazon every day? she asks.

Yes.

Doesn't he tell you he loves you all the time?

Yes.

Has he actually stopped texting you altogether?

No.

Is it possible that everything is fine?

Yes.

Do you still feel like you will keep spiralling?

Yes.

We talk now about the tyranny of expectational fields, of learned behaviour. The thing about the cycle is that even once you are aware of it, even once you are consciously trying to break free, to unlearn, the instinct is still there, and it is stubborn. So stubborn, in fact, that it has the power to project itself onto new people who are in fact being very present and loving. It twists their casual words into subtle goodbyes and their brief silences into abandonment. You put the belief out in the world so strongly that it becomes a lens through which you interpret everything, even the behaviour of those you have connected with precisely because they do not fit the mould. But it doesn't take long for the brain to remould them, cast upon them the very same thoughts and feelings as all the others, so those projected feelings can be cast back onto ourselves. How exhausting.

My therapist told me I struggle deeply with distrusting myself and my interpretation of the world. She was right: I am trapped in an endless cycle of not knowing whether I am projecting danger onto those who are safe or projecting safety onto those who are dangerous. When I feel the most strongly about something is when I doubt the truth of it the most, for the simple reason that it has come from my own mind.

Every single time I have believed something good about someone I have been wrong, I said when my therapist asked me what I was thinking.

.   .   .

Pema and I have already been speaking over Instagram for months by the time we finally meet at her house in North London. She has said she is willing to talk to me about her body, for my book, and so on a mild autumn day I wander to her house and knock, in the way you do when you feel like you know someone but you don't actually know them.

She opens the door and smiles widely, ushering me inside. She is taller than me, but she is dwarfed by the beautiful arched doorway she is standing in. It's my step-grandparents' house, she says as she notices me looking around. I'm just staying here while they're away.

She offers me a cup of tea and I accept, and one of us, I don't remember which, makes a joke about Australia, where we are both from. Her Perth accent is comforting to me. We are both so far from home. We talk about why she moved here, why I did. Then she inhales and says: Where should I start?

How about the beginning? I reply.

When Pema was nine, her parents moved her and her sister from their home on Australia's west coast to Ireland for three months. She didn't know it at the time, but the trip was a last-ditch attempt to save her parents' marriage. It didn't work.

Pema's mother was born in a small town in India, but her family was Tibetan. Her family fled Tibet after the CCP invasion and settled in India. She lived in the mountains and went to school in a mountainside building from which she could see her home.

By the time she was in her early twenties, she was working in a hospital and was engaged as part of an arranged marriage.

But then she met a doctor who had come to India from Australia to work in the hospital. They fell in love and Pema's mother broke off her engagement, moving back to Perth with the doctor.

They married soon after they arrived together in Australia – and just hours before Pema was born in a Perth hospital.

When Pema was ten, the couple split up.

Pema met Pete when she was seventeen. The two went to the same school in Perth, and they had a whirlwind, teenage relationship. Her father had remarried by this time, and Pema and her younger sisters had barely seen or heard from their mother in five years. She was back in Tibet.

One day, her mother had taken Pema aside and said: I think I need to leave. I just can't look after you or your sisters any more. I think I would be happier if I left. Do you think I should?

Swallowing all of her disappointment, Pema did what she had always been taught to do. She morphed into the adult in the situation. Yes, Mum, I think you should leave, she said. And that's what her mother did. When they had this conversation, Pema was twelve.

Both her father and stepmother seemed to like Pete. He was always polite when he came over for dinner, would always ask them how their day was.

During high school, Pema had always struggled with the way the other kids talked and jeered about her racial identity. Being mixed-race, Pema was never quite sure how to categorize herself, and it seemed that this was very important when all the kids around her started talking about sex and dating. She found that she constantly had to defend herself against assumptions about her as an Asian woman. And, she tells me, it was an introduction into her experience of being Asian in relationships: she was frequently gaslighted, stereotyped and erased.

But attraction felt easy with Pete, and she trusted that he liked her. Or at least, she tells me, she trusted that he needed her. They started talking about sex a few months into their relationship, started thinking about whether they should do it or not. Neither of them had had sex before, and they were both nervous, but especially Pema.

I was constantly worried about unwanted pregnancy, she tells me when we meet in 2019. I would think about it all the time, the worries would just spin around and around in my head and make me panic for hours, it would keep me up at night.

She also used to worry a lot about sexually transmitted infections. This became a major health anxiety, and she hated the thought of some invisible predator entering her body without her knowledge or permission.

She shared all of these anxieties with Pete, and he seemed to understand. He agreed to wait a bit longer so Pema could do some more research about how safe condoms were and what else she could do to protect her teenage body from the dangers of sex. Could you still get pregnant if you used a condom? Could you still get an infection? What should she do after the sex was over to reduce the risk of pregnancy?

Once she felt comfortable with the research she'd done, she told Pete she was ready.

They were at her house in West Perth while her father and stepmother were out. Pema was trying hard to keep her anxieties out of her mind. She knew, from hearing boys her age talk, that they all seemed to have an aversion to condoms. They all joked about how it didn't feel as good, that it just wasn't the same. But this confused her, because it seemed utterly reckless to have sex without condoms, so she didn't see an alternative. But she was hyper-aware that Pete might feel let down, like he'd missed out on something important and formative in that skin-on-skin contact, even that he might go and look for it somewhere else. But still, she insisted he wear one, and he agreed.

The sex hurt Pema quite a lot, but she also enjoyed the thrill of it. She felt so close to Pete, and he was whispering such sweet things in her ear, asking her if she was okay every few minutes, and she loved how joined-up they felt in those moments.

But something stopped Pema, an anxiety. She stopped him and glanced down. Panic sliced through her like glass.

Pete, where is the condom? Pema asked.

A pause.

Oh, it got too uncomfortable, so I took it off right after we started.

A hot flush of shame came out of nowhere, then terror. Pema leaped out of bed as though the sheets had electrocuted her and found herself cowering in a corner on the opposite side of the room, naked and afraid.

Woah woah woah, Pete said. What's wrong?

She spluttered and could barely get the words out.

Pete, you knew... you knew how scared I was. How could you do that?

Oh, I figured it was just silly anxiety in the build-up to it, and that you wouldn't mind it in the moment. And see, look, you didn't even notice!

Pema's mouth opened and closed and opened again. She could not believe what she was hearing. Did he really believe what he was saying?

But the thought was interrupted as Pema's insides started to shake, and she grabbed a towel and ran to the bathroom and vomited, hoping that the baby he might have deceptively inseminated her with would end up in the toilet.

Now, in her living room, Pema tells me that since that night when she was raped by her first boyfriend, she has found relationships difficult.

I'm always looking for a trapdoor, she says. A way out. She tells me that trust feels impossible sometimes.

Pema is a writer, and she has written about this night three times. The first in a letter to the boyfriend, her rapist. The second for her university literary magazine. The third for a magazine about illness, disability, pain and consent.

Pema wanted to speak right away about how hurt she felt, but she didn't have the words. Then one day, during her university years, she came across an academic article about the practice of 'stealthing': where men or people with penises covertly remove or break a condom after consent has been given on the condition of the use of the condom. The article said stealthing was illegal and 'rape-adjacent'.

As soon as she read the article, Pema told her sister, who was sitting in the room with her, what had happened.

That was years ago now. We no longer consider stealthing to be 'rape-adjacent'. It is rape. A landmark German case in 2019 determined that non-consensual condom removal is a form of rape, and convicted a police officer of the crime.

Other jurisdictions have followed suit. In November 2019, a Bournemouth man was found guilty of non-consensually removing a condom during sex and was sentenced to twelve years in prison.

The article Pema had read that day was by Alexandra Brodsky for the *Columbia Journal of Gender and Law*. Brodsky later told *HuffPost* that women were 'struggling with forms of mistreatment by sexual partners that weren't considered part of the recognized repertoire of gender-based violence – but that seemed rooted in the same misogyny and lack of respect'.

Stealthing was made illegal in the UK in 2017.

Returning to her story, Pema tells me that she crawled into the corner of the room and froze. At first Pete said nothing. Then he said sorry. He tried to touch her but she wouldn't let him. She just kept crying. Then he got angry and dismissive. He left her there, and she cried in the corner all night.

She stayed with him for another year after that, she says, and she doesn't know why. I was ashamed, she says, that he had hurt me so much. My confidence and my sense of self started to break down, and I didn't feel like I could leave.

In her recent essay about her rape, 'Anonymous', Pema writes:

Things began to dissolve around me. And I couldn't understand why. I struggled to feel like I could trust people. I felt like my work was not important, that I was indulgent for wanting to write a PhD on literature. Meanwhile, my activist work fell away too. I was listless. I dropped out of my doctoral programme and moved to England.

. . .

As I read this, I think, Pema and I have that in common. We both felt disintegrated after trauma and we had to leave for a new place, a new map. We might never have met if we'd stayed in Australia, but we had both left for similar reasons and had ended up only ten minutes away from each other in London.

Months later, she was working at a bar in Dalston. She turned up to her shift after spending hours watching Christine Blasey Ford testify about the night that then-Supreme Court nominee Brett Kavanaugh had raped her in 1987. When she arrived at work, she found she couldn't even look at the men she worked with. I hated all of them, she said.

Pema writes beautifully about her rape, and I can see the strength it takes when she talks to me about it. But she has done it. She writes about how men on message boards brag about stealthing, talk about how they want to covertly 'spread the seed'. That refers to semen, of course, but the practice also takes place in cis–gay relationships, so it's more than that. 'The seed is the leaving-behind of a physical and emotional legacy,' she says in her essay.

'Stealthing,' Pema writes, 'like other varieties of rape, is a way to ensure that you will always have a presence in a person's life. That you might retain a degree of power over them long after your personal relationship is over.'

This is how Pema's story ends: 'I wasn't murdered. I wasn't left with bruises, or with a broken wrist, or with any external wounds. I didn't receive any sexually transmitted infections or diseases, and I didn't become pregnant. I was just left adrift.'

When Pema talks about hating the men at her shift that day after watching the Blasey Ford testimony, I think about something Hannah Gadsby says in her comedy special *Nanette*. She says she is always accused of hating men.

I don't hate men, she says.

I don't hate men, but I am afraid of men.

And if you think a woman can stand in a room full of men without feeling moments of fear, Gadsby says, you aren't listening to the women in your life.

. . .

The more I progress through this book and the more I try and write about adulthood, the more I find myself coming back to childhood. The girl body is such a formative place.

. . .

I think it's remarkable when I speak to Sam, who is now twenty-nine and lives in Wales, that we have so many of the same ideas and feelings about sex and relationships. When she tells me about her intimate life, the thoughts she expresses strike me as though they could have come from my own brain. But when we dig deeper, I realize it's not the thoughts we have in common, it's their cause.

Sam grew up in the outskirts of cities in Spain, Portugal and the UK. She never stayed in one place very long, never had anywhere in particular to call home. She was part of a traveller community, living in trucks and caravans and teepees and never settling anywhere.

In the 1990s, Sam's parents were hosting a festival for their travelling community at a campsite in Spain. Sam's mother was heavily pregnant. As the summer light dwindled above the campsite and the festivalgoers started dragging their heavy feet to their caravans, Sam was born in an open field.

Homeschooled until she was fifteen, Sam did not grow up thinking about her body the way other teenage girls did. She did not have classmates or peers, only her sisters and the few other children at whatever campsite they had stopped at, but she never kept friends for long because her life was so transient.

When Sam was seven, she and her mother and her sisters moved to a caravan park in Spain. It was around this time that her mother became very ill with ME – also known as chronic fatigue syndrome – and found it difficult to take care of both Sam and herself. Without much of a support network, the little family began to struggle. Sam's mother had very little energy to care for a seven-year-old, so Sam found herself feeling very lonely and bored. She hadn't connected with any of the other children at the campsite, and she and her sisters felt isolated and alone.

After a few weeks, a British man in his fifties started chatting to Sam in the mornings as he sipped coffee in the park's communal area. Soon after that, he started taking her on walks around the campsite, talking to her about his life as a traveller, asking her about hers. They became close quite quickly, and Sam trusted him. She liked his company, and she liked having an adult who was so keen on paying attention to her.

So it didn't seem concerning to the little girl when Henry started asking her to have their talks inside his caravan rather than out strolling in the woods. Within a few months, he was reading aloud from pornographic magazines, explaining the concepts to her, talking about sex and sexuality for hours at a time while describing graphic sexual acts. Sam felt uncomfortable, but she didn't know why. Mostly, she was just confused. He would read from the magazines while pacing up and down the living room of the cramped caravan, asking her to watch as his penis became more and more erect.

One day, when Sam arrived in Henry's caravan, he said that he was feeling unwell. Inextricably close to him by this point in their relationship, Sam was immediately worried. She did not like their interactions, but she had come to depend on him so thoroughly. He cared about her.

But, he said, he would be all right as long as Sam agreed to be his nurse. She nodded her head furiously.

From that day on, Henry would get naked when Sam arrived in his caravan and would ask her to rub olive oil all over his body, saying it would heal him if she did it every day. He would lie down on his back and ask the small girl to straddle his stomach and rub the oil over his middle-aged body.

Not long after that, he started asking her to kiss his erect penis while he watched.

While the abuse was taking place, Sam never spoke a word about it to anyone. Most likely because she did not have a word for it – the word 'abuse' would not come into her mind until years and years later. Sam and her mother and her sisters moved away from the site in Spain, so thousands of miles were quickly put between her and Henry. She tried as hard as she could to forget about him, and most days it worked.

A few years later, Sam's family moved to a Welsh town and made a home in a new caravan park outside the town centre. When Sam was nine, she was doing the weekly grocery shopping with her sisters at the local supermarket when out of the corner of her eye she spotted a man who looked like Henry. This had happened a few times over the years since they had left Spain, so Sam had grown used to correcting the false positive sightings of him when the men drew closer and turned out to be any old middle-aged punters.

But not this time. This *was* Henry. And he was walking towards her.

Sam, he said cheerily. It's me, Henry! Remember me?

Sam found herself unable to speak. She opened and closed her mouth, but no words came out.

From the campsite in Spain! he said, grinning from ear to ear. She stayed silent, so he continued, It's so wonderful to see you again!

More pressing than the need to form words in her mouth was Sam's confusion about how a coincidence like this could possibly have occurred.

Her nine-year-old brain just kept thinking about how far away they felt from Spain, how different Wales was, how she had adapted to a new language and new people and new places a number of times between Spain and this supermarket. He couldn't have followed them, they'd moved around so many times since then. How on earth could it be that he was now standing here, in the vegetable aisle of an impossibly small Welsh town that no one had ever heard of?

As if reading her mind, or perhaps just reading her silence, Henry started speaking again.

I remember when I used to chat to your mum back at the campsite. She would always mention this town as somewhere she might move to when you girls were older, when she was thinking about sending you to school. So I visit here every so often, just to see if I can find you.

Sam's stomach turned to stone and her throat closed up even more. She took a step back towards where her sisters were standing and then started walking away. Instinctively they followed.

The family stayed in Wales, moving from town to town, for a few years after that. At fifteen, Sam would eventually be enrolled in a Welsh college to take her A levels.

She continued her project of trying not to think or talk about Henry. She mentioned it to her mother once, but she saw immediately that her mother could not bear the news, could not carry the weight of it. Feeling instantly guilty, feeling that shame she had felt as a child trying to wrest away her mother's attention when she had so little of it to give, she finished the conversation as quickly as she could, and neither of them brought it up again after that.

During those years of high school, Sam found a diary from that year in Spain. She clenched up as she read her messy, seven-year-old handwriting describing the man who used to 'make her touch his willy'.

Around this same time, Sam started having nightmares about strange men climbing into her bedroom through her window, or reaching in through the window and pulling her out, plucking her from her bed where she lay, where she thought she was safe.

.   .   .

I don't hate men, but I am afraid of men, I think as Sam tells me this story.

It was a man who sexually abused me as a child, Gadsby says in *Nanette*. It was a man who attacked me at a bus stop. It was two men who raped me in my twenties.

.   .   .

I fire up my laptop and open Zoom. I am scheduled to speak to a woman named Tay, who I adore the moment her face pops up on my screen. We smile big smiles at each other.

Tay opened up her copy of her Greek newspaper recently, she tells me, the one she still reads to remind her of home, and found a review of a novel that had just been published in Greece by one of her close friends. She smiled, snapped a photo of the review and sent it to her friend. Her friend replied, thanking her, and then said: Ha, isn't that that guy we went to university with?

Tay scanned the page, and to the left of her friend's book was another, shorter review. This one was of a novel that had just been published by a man they had known at university. A man Tay had been flirtatious with at one point in her life.

I need to stop being attracted to solipsistic men who write books, Tay says to me now, laughing, and I nod furiously in agreement. Me too, I say.

Then Tay's face shifts, and she says: I feel like this might be a good place to start my story.

At university, Tay and her friends were studying English literature in Athens. She had a good, supportive group of friends and she enjoyed her university life. The man who went on to write the novel would often flirt with her in class and around campus. She would flirt back, in that way you do sometimes, but nothing ever happened and they both knew it never would. It was just one of those things.

One night, the group was having a house party and Tay accidentally got very drunk. I nod furiously again when she says this to me – it happens to me all the time. Especially with wine.

So Tay was drunk and her friend, who was hosting the party, suggested she sleep there to make sure she didn't have to navigate the dark streets at that hour. But then the soon-to-be novelist came over and said, Don't worry, I'll drive her home. Tay was told this later; she doesn't remember much of the conversation first-hand.

The next time Tay was aware of herself, she was in his car and he was on top of her, kissing her, with his hands all over her body. She came back into consciousness with a start and she panicked, not knowing how she had ended up in his car or why he was assaulting her.

She got out of the car, got into bed and tried not to think about that night again. It came to her mind once or twice, but she pushed it away. She didn't properly think about it again until years later, when she was speaking to a friend from home who ended up dating this man, the novelist, for a short period. The friend spoke to her in whispers, confessing that he had done some very uncomfortable things to her, made her feel coerced. Tay's eyes widened and she nodded and said: Me too.

Violence against women in Greece is very difficult to talk about, Tay tells me. It is so pervasive, so mundane, that it doesn't really have its own language. The culture does not hold within it the recognition we are now developing in some parts of the world about the long-term implications of violence, and gendered violence in particular.

I was never, ever able to view any of the things that happened to me as violence, Tay tells me. Because in Greek, I just didn't have the words. I was so convinced that everything was my fault, that I had asked for it, that I deserved it.

This is not, of course, to say that the UK has a perfect – or even a better – approach to violence, Tay says. It's just different. Here, when I speak in English, I have the words.

I am struck when Tay tells me that she still cannot say the word *rape* in Greek, even though she is now comfortable using that word to describe her experience in English. She knows what it is now, she says. But she cannot say the Greek word. It feels too violent in that language, too strong in her mouth, because of the linguistic and cultural associations it carries. Also, she tells me, she cannot bear to use the language of her childhood to represent that night.

A few years later, Tay was struck down again and again by bouts of anxiety and depression, uncontrollable moods that haunted her. She started seeing a psychologist to try and cope. She also started self-medicating. Alcohol, drugs. Anything to make her feel better. Eventually, a trusted therapist would give her a tentative diagnosis of type II bipolar disorder, but he was reluctant to give her a formal diagnosis because, according to this therapist, the only recognized treatment is a sometimes lifelong course of lithium. He helped Tay focus on different symptoms she could try and manage on her own, and together they got a handle on things.

Tay moved from her home town of Athens to an English city to study for her PhD in poetry and gender. She hoped to turn her thesis on revolutionary poets into a book and then into an academic career. When she first arrived, she was excited about the prestigious institution she was joining. But it wasn't long before she met Jake, an older man who was also studying for a PhD in her department.

He was a good guy, Tay tells me. So when he claimed that everything that happened later was because I was some hyper-aroused Mediterranean sexual animal, when he said he couldn't help himself, everyone believed him, she says, with resignation in her voice and all over her face. There were so many times when I said no and he forced himself on me. I cried, I said no, I went silent. Eventually I gave in. I was supposed to want it.

At the beginning of their courtship, Jake was unsure about Tay. They went home together a few nights after university events, but he didn't think he wanted a relationship. He was holding back, so she held on tighter.

One night, Tay brought Jake back to his flat because he was drunk at a pub quiz and needed help getting home. He had said again and again that he didn't want to be with her, so she planned on putting him into bed and leaving him there. But he protested, begged her to stay, offered to pay for her cab the next morning if she just slept beside him, and she thought: This is the first time I have felt truly wanted by him.

After that night, they started dating properly. Jake had a big flat to himself near the university, so they would always go to his house to avoid Tay's flatmates. He would often go into work for the day and ask her to stay there, in his flat, until he got home. She thought: This is how much he trusts me with his belongings.

Their relationship became more and more and more insular. They would spend days holed up in his flat, him coming and going, her staying indoors. Her friends started to say they did not like the way he spoke to her in public, at university events and at the pub. She waved it away.

There is something so potent about someone who withholds themselves from you so completely, who pulls away each time you step closer. It's like magic: as soon as they are willing to put up with any amount of closeness, they suddenly have the power to do whatever they want with you.

In that flat, they would go for whole afternoons without speaking when Jake would decide he was angry at her about something. She would speak and he would ignore her, over and over again. Then he would climb onto the bed where she was reading and grab on to her body, coaxing her to have sex with him, returning to silence when he had finished.

Whenever she thought about the sex she felt coerced into, Tay felt hot shame come over her. He never even wanted to be with me, she would think. I was the one who wanted him. So how can I now claim that he wants me so much he cannot take no for an answer? Who would believe me?

This had been going on for a few months the first time he hit her. They were in the middle of an argument, and out of nowhere he swung a closed fist towards her. His knuckles connected with her eye socket, and she fell back on the couch behind her.

That wasn't the only time she had sex with Jake when she didn't want to. It kept happening. The relationship became more and more intense, which was confusing because in some ways that's what Tay had wanted when he was being so distant and unattainable.

He would invite her over on a Monday night and she would wake up on Friday and realize he'd convinced her to stay all week. When he would leave for the day to teach or to get some work done at the university, she would start getting dressed and he would say, No, no, why don't you stay here for the day? And she would say, No, it's okay, I need to go home and get some clothes, and he would say, Oh, looking downcast, and then say, But it feels so nice when you stay at my house when I'm not here, it makes it feel like we're a real couple, like we live together. And when he said that, she would have that same thought she had during sex: This is what I wanted. I wanted more of him. I wanted more *from* him. How can I complain when I get it?

So with those thoughts swirling around in her head, thoughts about selfishness and gratitude, she would stay. She began to notice that he would always take the keys to the flat with him, so she would be locked inside all day, able to eat only what was left in his fridge. When she asked to have the keys with her, he would say: Where do you need to go? And she would say, Nowhere in particular, just in case I need to go to the shop, and he would say, Just tell me what you need and I'll get it for you on the way home, and then he would close the door behind him, keys in hand.

Sitting in that flat all day, with nowhere to go and no one to see, Tay would swing violently between happiness and dread. She would wonder how she had lost her sense of reality, of what was right and what was wrong for her.

It's funny, isn't it, she says to me now, over Zoom. Looking back, I definitely had doubts. All those days locked in the flat, I questioned whether he was abusive. I knew, somewhere, that he was. Some unconscious part of me knew the truth, but I kept talking myself out of it. I wanted this. *I wanted this*.

But when he punched me, it's like a fog was lifted, she tells me. Everything became clearer after that. I started to look back on everything else that had happened in the lead-up to that, and it all became clearer. I started to see all the little things he had done to control me. All the nasty things he said. All the put-downs, all the times he locked me in his flat. Maybe that sounds crazy, she says.

It doesn't, I say, and I mean it. It makes perfect sense to me.

And then, after a pause, she says: Isn't that crazy? The fact that I was so certain that the only valid act of abuse was physical violence that I ignored everything else until that moment?

It is, I say. It's criminal, the way we are told there is a red line that exists right after the moment he throws the first punch. Before that, we think we have no good reason to leave.

Tay nods. I wish there were more public conversations about emotional abuse and coercive control, she says, and I agree with her. If there were, Tay adds, maybe I would have seen the signs. Because without those explicit conversations, all we have to go on is our experiences. And all of our experiences tell us one, fundamental thing: it could be worse.

So Tay's brain connected Jake's controlling behaviour to the novelist in the car and she assumed that because he had never done anything openly threatening like that, she should feel like it was okay. This is how being a woman works. Everything is relative, and the worst things women have experienced are so much worse than anyone thinks. In comparison, everything else is manageable. The reason women never get over their formative traumas is because they become weapons with which they excuse and allow all the others, all the more insidious violations that follow. It's not just that first act of violence, but all the ones it opens doors to. All the ones it hides.

Tay stayed with Jake for a few more months after he hit her that first time. There was more violence, physical and sexual, but she felt as though she ought to give it a few more chances. When she finally left the relationship, she had to leave the university too, she tells me. Because she and Jake were members of the same department, and because he was everywhere, and because he had convinced her friends he was a good guy, and because everyone believed him. Almost everyone in their group of friends had taken his side. Whether that was because they really believed him when he accused her of lying, or because they wanted to remain close to the power he held in a hallowed academic institution that thrived on hierarchy, she didn't know.

I will probably never know, she tells me. But I do know that I saw all those people in my group at the next women's march, holding signs that said BELIEVE ALL WOMEN. But what about me?

A few months after she finally left Jake, Tay was visiting her home town in Greece and met a man named Jean. He was handsome and charming, and seemed kind. They clicked immediately. He lived in Athens and she still lived in the UK, so they started a long-distance relationship that was intensely loving and seemed to both of them to have long-term potential.

Tay flew back to Greece often to see him, and they had a beautiful honeymoon period. It was a few months before he started saying things that made her uncomfortable. Backhanded compliments, the occasional hurtful, poisonous remark. By then she had met his parents, and she felt happy that things were progressing.

But as time went on, she started feeling things that were familiar from her time with Jake. Jean would be emotionally intense one week and completely withdrawn the next. She never knew what to expect from him, which was particularly hard when they lived so far away and had to conduct most of their relationship on WhatsApp. She started to realize that her own emotions were being thrown around wildly by his behaviour, and it made her feel unstable and needy. He started being crueller and crueller, until one day she asked him to talk.

I'll come and see you at work, he said. I'm in London this week.

They met up and he was charming again, very kind and loving, and she immediately felt better. They arranged for her to go to Athens the following weekend so they could spend a romantic weekend together.

But later that afternoon, he texted her from the airport: I can't do this. I can't deal with your emotions.

And she never saw or heard from him again.

. . .

Why did I fall for it this time? she asks me.

Because we all do, I say, because that's how it works. Because abuse takes our agency away, forces us to keep coming back to the same lessons again and again and again. Because it wasn't as bad as the last time. Because we are drawn to what we know. Because of expectational fields.

I don't hate men, I think, *but I am afraid of men.*

And that's not irrational or hypersensitive. Neither is Sam's fear of dark windows or Pema's fear of trust or Tay's fear of relationships. These are rational responses to the evidence we have all collected. The fear response is constructed out of our concepts, our memories, and those things are tarnished.

Emotional abuse, like physical abuse, causes a victim to distrust themselves. By creating an environment inside the relationship where thoughts, behaviour and reactions are unpredictable and chaotic, the abuser causes us to question what we know about the world. If we have grown up knowing that certain behaviour leads to kindness, or safety, or reward, and then all of a sudden that same behaviour leads to anger, and shame, and stonewalling, and violence, we automatically believe we, and not our partners, are wrong about how people are supposed to behave.

Do you remember when I told you, earlier in the book, that when we are young and people abuse us, we are unable to fathom that an adult could be bad or dysfunctional so we assume that we are the cause of the problem? That we are bad and cause certain adults to behave badly around us? The same thing happens in relationships. If we live with chronic shame, and we end up with emotionally abusive partners, we already have a belief that we are toxic or rotten, so we immediately believe that it is us that is causing the problem and that the abuser is just coping as best they can with our deficiencies.

Pema said, Why did I stay? Tay said, Why did I fall for it again? The answer is simple. Because shame is a trap. When Pema's boyfriend got angry and defensive about her reaction to the sexual assault, he started a process of making her believe that her world was not real. Jake and Jean did the same to Tay. Shame is the glue that holds the false world together.

Once, I broke up with someone after a sustained pattern of emotional abuse. It was so difficult to leave him, but finally I did. I had started to notice that the internal world of our relationship was skewed. That the things he said were unforgivable about me were actually just human. That his chaos was a prison for me. In other words, I started to fly out of the bottle.

I finally broke up with him, and a few days later we met up in a park in Sydney.

He said, I know you want this to work, but I think it's over for me.

He said, I'm sorry.

He said, I know how hard this is for you.

A few months earlier I would have believed it. That really, it was him who left. That really, he still had the power.

But on that day, I didn't think that at all. I remember so clearly looking out at the park, at the people playing with their dogs and getting drunk with their friends and kissing on swing sets and I thought:

That, out there, is the real world. This, what he's constructing between him and me, is a fiction.

After years of being shamed in relationships, I often find myself with the distinct impression that I am sliding between two worlds. Like I am slippery, stuck in some liminal space between reality and someone else's narrative.

Every week, my therapist and I have some version of the following conversation:

Sometimes I think I know something, I say, and then I see something and it makes me question everything, and then I think, I don't know what's real.

And she says, I think you do. I think you do know.

The liminal space is closing, and I am moving into surer footing in the real world.

CHAPTER EIGHT

I never really came out publicly as bisexual. I think I always knew it on some level. I experimented with it in high school, but I always felt afraid of that part of myself. Mostly, I fantasized about women while alone at home, scrolling through pictures of beautiful girls I wanted to know everything about.

I didn't actually embrace this part of myself until I was twenty-six. I had just come out of a long-term relationship with a man, and I spent almost every weeknight endlessly swiping through Tinder and Bumble, thinking about how I had exploded my life and I would have to start all over again. I kept thinking: Maybe now is the time to try and date women. And then I would think, No, no, not yet, not now, no.

I have unbelievably supportive friends – something that is a godsend for so many queer people, most of whom have had a much more difficult time than me – and the more I started thinking about dating women, the more it started slipping out of me during lunches with those closest to me.

I have one friend who knows about my trouble with relationships with men, my trouble with sex. She is one of those friends everybody wishes for – she is there to cheer you on at every bright moment, no matter how hard it is for her to be there. She is always there on the other end of the phone when things are bad, too. She and I worked together, so we spent every day together. She helped me so much to wiggle my way out of my last relationship, so she knows how afraid I am of sex. How much I hate being touched.

So it seemed right that it was also her who I told first about my rape. She dropped me home one day, just a few days after I had disclosed my rape to my doctors and therapists. We were talking about banal things – work, life, the meal we had had near her flat.

But then suddenly, I just said it. I told her everything. And she hugged me, and she held my hand, and the next three years of my life, I think, were set in motion in that moment.

I don't mean to talk about my rape when I'm talking about my sexuality. Or maybe I do. But the point is, this friend asked me one night: Do you think you could be gay?

What I thought was: How did she see into my soul?

But what I said was: I've been thinking about this so much.

What I said next was: I'm not gay, no. I know that. But I am bisexual. I know that too. I've been trying to work myself up to dating women.

And from that moment onwards, she would visit my desk and swipe through girls' profiles with me on Tinder, on Bumble, she helped me craft those first messages to girls trying to explain to them: I know I am queer, but I've spent years in a relationship with a man. I need you to know that, because it's okay if you don't want to go on a date. I don't want you to feel used or experimented on, I said.

In the days after that, I kept deleting and re-downloading the apps, because I was scared of what I had done. But slowly, I stopped, and I started having real conversations with women on them, and I started going on dates. And it was amazing.

·   ·   ·

When Rowan first started losing weight, she tells me it was because she wanted to look androgynous. She knew this in her heart, but she wouldn't have admitted it out loud at the time. She wanted to rid herself of her most womanly features. That's why, she tells me, being in hospital during inpatient treatment for her eating disorder was so excruciating for her. Forced to put on so much weight so quickly, she had to watch a woman's body grow underneath her, in a single hospital bed, a body she didn't want.

It wasn't until after Rowan came out of hospital that she properly realized she was gay. Dating and romance felt almost impossible in her new, bigger body, so she didn't act on her feelings for a while. But eventually, she worked up the courage to join a dating website for lesbians. That's where she met Nicole. They are still dating when we speak in 2020, and Rowan grins from ear to ear when she talks about her. They are forced to have a long-distance relationship because Nicole is still in London and Rowan is in Birmingham, but they make it work.

When we are talking about Nicole, Rowan says something that stays with me.

I'm still recovering, she says. I will always be recovering. So many of us are recovering from something. So I hate it when I see those Instagram posts that say 'you can't love anyone else until you love yourself'. That's not true, she says. That puts too much pressure on us to love ourselves. Loving ourselves is constant, everyday work. It is never finished. I am still learning to love myself, and it is gruelling. I'm not good at it yet. But that doesn't mean I am incapable of love. I have so much love to give.

I love hearing Rowan say this. It speaks to everything I have noticed about her since she became an interview subject for this book. Most of all, it speaks to her bravery. She won't let anyone tell her that she isn't able to love, no matter how much she has had to live through. The worst years of her life won't define her. She will always be recovering, and she might never totally accept herself, but she is still here, and she is going to make the most of it by pouring her love into others until she has enough for herself. I respect that mightily.

·   ·   ·

I am scared to write these pages because I am scared I do not know enough about queerness to write about it. I am scared I do not have the authority, because I've spent so long in different-gender relationships. And the truth is that I do not have the experience of growing up visibly queer, and until my mid-twenties I was completely sheltered from any of the public abuse or discrimination that queer people have to live with. In that regard, I *am* completely inexperienced, and I will never pretend not to be.

But here is what I know about my bisexuality. It is real even though there were times in my life when I didn't express it. It is a valuable and important part of me. My romantic attraction to women has always defined me, even before I could explore it in real life and not just alone in my bedroom.

And here's what else I know. I have never felt more comfortable than on dates with women – whether they are first dates, fourth dates or date nights at home after months of being in a relationship. I do not feel gaslighted or ashamed or un-whole. I feel seen and understood.

I am not, of course, saying these things don't happen in queer relationships. I have purposefully included a story about emotional abuse in a queer relationship in this book because my own experiences have been very positive. These dynamics can play out in any relationship, I know that. I just haven't experienced that yet. So far, my small amount of experience of dating women has been extremely enriching.

. . .

Rachel met her first girlfriend online and they fell in love quickly. They spent their entire year out from school together, falling more and more in love, and Rachel thought she was happy.

The sex they had was experimental and fun, and Rachel was comfortable in the knowledge that queer sex – its inclusivity, its discursive quality – was what she wanted. When Rachel tells me this story, it feels like it is playing in Technicolor in my mind, a montage of the kind of safe and explorative sex I desperately want teenage girls to have. But like any story in this book, and like any story of womanhood, it does not end there.

Rachel's partner quickly became the most extreme version of herself in all things. She started expecting Rachel to try all manner of things during sex that Rachel wasn't comfortable with. She never pushed her to do anything she didn't want to, but Rachel started feeling guilty about the fact that they weren't on the same page. As their intimacy became murkier and more distant, Rachel's girlfriend started withholding sex in a way that hurt Rachel deeply.

Sex became an incredibly hostile, thorny endeavour. Rachel couldn't understand what had gone wrong, and she wanted to try and fix it. But every time she initiated sex she was turned down, and sometimes her girlfriend would initiate physical intimacy only to pull away and, Rachel thought, intentionally make her feel repulsive and rejected.

By the time Rachel left their home town to go to university, the two had stopped having sex altogether. But her partner had started pulling closer in other, more destructive ways. She was poring over all of Rachel's bank statements to make sure she wasn't buying gifts for other people. She was reading her mail and her text messages and her emails. Rachel felt trapped, and far too afraid to speak up.

Rachel left for university and started making new friends who made her feel animated again, far from the girl she had become at home. Her girlfriend became more and more possessive, though, and got her into trouble when she went out during Freshers' week or to bars after lectures.

Rachel started feeling more and more out of control about her own life, and her destructive eating habits started gnawing at the edge of her brain. This is something I noticed with almost every single person I spoke to for this book – there is something so permanent about the regime of restriction, it stays with us, ready to be deployed at any moment we need to start hurting ourselves again. The calorie-counters in our heads are never forgotten, never retired, only put on a shelf until they are needed, and we can call on them whenever we feel that urge to self-punish.

Rachel felt isolated and alone at university because she couldn't spend time with her friends and because she missed the physical intimacy she had once had with her partner. Eventually, in the summer after first year, she found the courage to drive to her girlfriend's house and end the relationship.

It seems so strange to say, she tells me when we meet in 2020, but I really just blossomed after that day.

When I speak to Rachel, she is twenty-three and completing a master's in modern history at university. She tells me all about her thesis, which I desperately want to read. It is about inherited trauma – the way in which traumatic events are passed down through generations, in our bones and our blood.

Speaking to Rachel now, I am astonished by her. She is brilliant and articulate and clever. I am enamoured with her – I can tell that she blossomed after that day.

.   .   .

I am not afraid of women. I am not afraid of being close to them. I am not afraid of being seen by them. I trust them with myself.

Sex with women is a genuinely positive experience. Not pleasurable, precisely – I think there is a part of me that is so afraid of that realm of existence that I suspect I will never experience sexual pleasure – but enjoyable, certainly. Loving, definitely. Open, always.

There is something about the communication involved in queer sex that I really, really love. There's no script in the way I have always felt there is with sex with men. In my experience, nothing has been expected of me, there is no role I am asked to fill. We just talk, we find out what the other person wants and doesn't, and we negotiate. That, to me, is real intimacy between lovers.

When I compare those experiences to sex with men – which I do still have, occasionally, but less and less so – it seems striking to me that I ever thought my own experience of heterosexual sex was intimate, or was an example of intimacy. It never was. It was so distant.

It stirred up shame in me because I was mostly voiceless, usually dispensable, and sometimes disrespected by the particular sexual scripts that men grow up with.

Because of all these things, it bolstered and reinforced my shame, it kept it on a loop, always returning to the scene of the crime. But sex with women doesn't, and I feel so lucky to be bisexual, to be able to access this sacred space. I will never take it for granted.

2

Two weeks to six months after:

- · Forgetfulness
- · Exhaustion
- · Guilt
- · Nightmares

CHAPTER NINE

I have been thinking a lot about retribution. What does it mean to want it, or to get it, or to have it?

It is so often assumed that we are seeking retribution when we try and hold people accountable for sexual abuse. That we want them to suffer, like we did. That we want people to hurt. But I don't think that's always the case. It's not what Cleo or Victoria or Riley wanted in the stories I'm about to tell you. It's not what I would have wanted if I'd ever gone to the police about my rape.

We all just want our own hurting to stop. We seek justice because the shame and the pain and the tears just keep coming, and coming, and coming, and the assaults bleed into every other relationship, into our own heads, into our families and friends and our diaries and our beliefs. We seek justice in a courtroom because we need to exorcize it somehow, we need to externalize it.

We don't want them to suffer, not really. Or I don't, at least. I just want them to stop.

I want accountability because I want these predators to change, not because I want them to hurt.

I want accountability because I want my own pain to stop.

What strikes me about Cleo and Riley and Victoria's testimonies is that their pain was exacerbated by the process of reporting to the police simply because no one properly acknowledged their experience of it. Because no one acknowledged what comes after. No one acknowledged that they didn't need revenge, they needed help. They needed someone to tell them that it was real, and that one day it would be over.

Most of all, we just want someone to tell us it was real, that it mattered, that this event lived a life inside our bodies. Only then can you let it go. For real acceptance to happen, something has to die. Before it dies you have to let it live. That's all we are asking for.

· · ·

Victoria was born in Melbourne to a white mother and a Ghanaian father. Her father left when she was very young and re-entered her life only sporadically, so she never really knew him. He was always a spectre in her life, a ghostly presence, but never a tangible one. Her mother rarely spoke about him.

Most of all, he was a ghost on her skin. A presence she could never ignore because it was etched into her biracial identity. It was pointed out to her almost every day in white, middle-class Melbourne. As much as she wanted to forget her father, she knew she never could. The world would not let her. No matter how far away he stayed, he showed up every day on her hands and face and legs and hair.

His absence from her life and her family meant that Victoria never learned much about her Ghanaian heritage or identity. The Black side of her was almost erased as she grew up because her mother knew little about it and her father wasn't around to teach it to her. Her father and his family all lived in Ghana, and she rarely got the chance to visit. She felt so deprived of this part of herself that she began to resent it, she told me.

Victoria always hated her body as a child and as a teenager. She hated being so much taller and darker than all the other girls in her school. She felt unattractive and unworthy. The boys she knew would always bring up her race when they teased her, as well as when they objectified her. Her neighbourhood was not very diverse, and as she grew older, she felt more and more alone.

Just after she finished high school, Victoria was scouted to become a model. This was because she was tall, the agency told her, and also, she suspected, because she was dark-skinned. She accepted the offer because it seemed to her a good way to try and accept the way she looked. Also, she tells me, she was a teenager, and being a model is something every teenage girl wants. I know what she means, I think. I used to dream of it myself.

But like anything that sharpens, feeds off and commodifies the objectification of women, the modelling industry proved much more damaging to Victoria than it was useful or productive. The body she had always hated suddenly became the focus of her life and her livelihood. Instead of helping her accept her body, the experience just made her hate it even more. And now she was less able to get away from it than ever. Like so many models, she went down a a path of destructive behaviours designed to break her body down, to punish it for causing her so much pain.

This was compounded by the fact that her racial identity had been put front and centre of all her modelling campaigns, although she still didn't understand what it meant to her. She still had no connection to her Ghanaian family, and it made her feel alien to herself.

At seventeen, not long after she started modelling, Victoria was gang-raped by two men while she was out with friends one night in Melbourne. It shattered her, she tells me. It changed everything.

I can tell from my conversations with Victoria that she is not prone to exaggeration; everything about her seems even-tempered. So when she says these words, I know she really means them. I can feel it in her voice, too.

After the rape Victoria left her body altogether, she says. She floated away, unable to bear the feeling of living inside it, unable to bear the reminders of the way she had been torn open in the night by two strange men.

Victoria is a very private person – this is another thing I can see clearly from our conversations. So for the next year she didn't tell anyone about her rape. She kept it to herself, without even thinking about it. Just like I had done ten years earlier. But about a year after the attack, Victoria found herself wanting to tell her mother. She and her mother were close, and she knew she would find some comfort in telling her. And eventually, she did.

Victoria's mother jumped to her defence immediately and wholly. She asked if Victoria would like to go to the police, and after giving it some thought, Victoria said yes, she would.

The process of reporting her rape to the police was gruelling and draining, but she got through it. She made statement after statement, and eventually the police arrested and charged her two attackers with sexual assault in the first degree.

She wondered how their conviction would make her feel, but ultimately this was in vain. She would never find out. The police eventually sat Victoria down and said there just wasn't enough evidence to pursue the prosecution, and that they had decided to drop the charges.

It's just your word against theirs, the cops said to her.

This breaks my heart when she relays it to me: that on some level, she wasn't believed.

Figures from the Office for National Statistics show that recorded rapes in the UK doubled between the financial years 2014–15 and 2018–19, to 58,614. In the year 2019–20 the Crown Prosecution Service completed charging decisions in relation to 4,184 suspects, and 1,867 (44.7%) of those suspects were charged. The frequency of rape, or at least its reporting, is increasing. But convictions are falling.

In 2019–20, 1,439 suspects in cases where a rape had been alleged were convicted of rape or another crime – half the number recorded this time three years ago, according to the CPS data summary for the fourth quarter of that year. The number of completed prosecutions in 'rape-flagged' cases was the lowest since tracking began in 2009.

Overall prosecutions – which include those that ended in acquittal – also peaked in 2016–17, with 5,190 completed cases, but the figures dropped to 2,102 in 2019–20.

Police forces in the UK, US and Australia continue to find hoards of untested rape kits – evidence collected from victims that is left to languish on a shelf, never tested, never looked at again – as reported, for example, by Tom Jackman in 'Funding for Untested Rape Kits and DNA Evidence Stalls in Congress' for the *Independent*.

Only one in sixty-five rape cases reported to police results in suspects being summonsed or charged, a *Guardian* analysis of the latest crime figures shows:

> The most recent Home Office statistics highlight an alarming decline in rape prosecutions in England and Wales over recent years amid increasingly acrimonious rows over the disclosure of evidence and suggestions that CPS prosecuting policies [have] changed.
>
> The drop is particularly dramatic at a time when victims are reporting more attacks. Four years ago, one in seven or 14% of cases led to a suspect being charged or summonsed – a total of 4,908 in 2015–16. Last year fewer than one in sixty-five reports of rape (1.5%) resulted in a charge or a summons, for a total of only 886 in 2018–19.

Some would say that as rape is being spotlighted for the rich and famous, it's being slowly decriminalized for the rest of us.

. . .

Cleo was twenty-four when she was sexually assaulted. What's more, she was a criminal defence lawyer. She had all the tools to take control of her situation and ensure a prosecution, but even for her the process was arduous and shattering.

She had graduated from law school and started her first proper job as a solicitor. The pay was bad, and the hours were long, but Cleo was okay with it because it was the job she wanted. She was working for a human rights lawyer who had worked on the kinds of cases young lawyers only ever dream of. The big ones. The ones that really make a difference to people's lives. Cleo didn't know it then, but soon enough she would be working on one of the highest-profile criminal cases in the country.

The office was understated and not overly comfortable, but Cleo didn't mind. She sat next to another young solicitor, who was only slightly more experienced than she was. He was friendly, and they chatted often throughout the day. But he was competitive, and only liked to take on cases he knew for sure he would win. This meant a lot of the scraps, the lost causes, ended up on Cleo's desk.

When we talk five years later, in 2020, Cleo tries to explain to me how unusual it is for a first-year lawyer to be managing cases on her own. But she doesn't need to – I trained as a lawyer too, and I know how those first few years so often look.

So I was very lucky, she says, a refrain that will repeat throughout her story again and again.

She had a boyfriend at the time, someone she had met four months before. They were getting along well and he was sweet, if a little distant.

Aren't they all, we both laugh over Zoom. (This is another thing that comes up again and again in my interviews for this book: how low we set our standards just to avoid disappointment.)

In the first month of her new job, Cleo went to a day spa near her house to try and relax her back and neck muscles, pounding as they were from many twelve-hour days in a row at the office. The massage really helped, she tells me one bright Friday morning (for me) and Friday evening (for her). She felt relaxed afterwards, and she had written down some of the massage therapist's advice to keep her muscles in check.

Work got more and more stressful. Cleo started work on a national inquiry into child sex abuse, deeply traumatizing cases that would follow her around for years. The job required her to travel to different parts of the country to interview witnesses and victims of institutional abuse that went unchecked for decades. She sat in small, dark rooms with the victims, now adults, an extra chair left for the ghosts of the children they used to be, the ones they were calling on to rehash the memories.

Sometimes Cleo had to represent perpetrators, which she struggled a great deal with. Unsure where or who to place her feelings with, she felt pressured and overworked. She found herself drinking heavily with the other lawyers working on the inquiry after long days in court.

It was a Saturday when Cleo scheduled another massage, keen to work the knots out of her forehead and stomach. She and her best friend used to give each other massage vouchers each year for their birthdays, and she had chosen this particular Saturday to cash in hers because she and her boyfriend were going to a house party later and she wanted to have just one night of feeling able to relax like a normal twenty-four-year-old.

When we get to this part of her story and Cleo says the name of the day spa in Sydney, I react instinctively. Ah! I say. I love that place. I used to go there once a month. I am smiling the kind of smile I reserve for those beautiful moments of feeling connected to someone who is far away, but I don't get the response I expect. Her face drops and she pauses. Sorry, go on, I say, conscious that I shouldn't have interrupted her.

Her voice is a little softer when she continues, telling me that she grinned widely as the massage therapist greeted her. He asked the usual questions: Why was she there? What would he like her to focus on?

She was standing right by the door to the small room. The man was standing in front of the massage table, leaning heavily, almost sitting on it. His legs were spread very wide, the kind of pose you would give a disapproving, sideways glance to on a train.

Cleo dutifully answered his questions, explaining that she was very stressed at work and would like him to focus on her neck and back. He left the room so that she could get changed and lie face down on the massage table.

When the man walked back in, he started on the back of her neck, as she had requested. But his fingers were ever so gentle. She could barely feel them. It was as though he was lightly grazing his fingers over her neck rather than massaging the knots out of it. Cleo had always preferred particularly vigorous massages, but she figured maybe he was just taking his time to get into the swing of things.

After her neck, he moved on to her leg muscles. She was about to ask him to use a bit more pressure, but something stopped her. It almost felt like the man was trying to be sensual, trying to be erotic in some way. He kept using more and more massage oil and moving his fingers lightly across her legs, pulling them all the way up towards her upper thigh.

Cleo froze. From that moment on, she said nothing.

His fingers grew closer and closer to her crotch with every movement. Then the man asked her to turn over so he could massage her front. She was terrified, her heart racing, but she did as she was told.

The man put the fresh white towel over her body and almost immediately put his hands underneath, massaging her breasts slowly and purposefully.

Do you know that feeling when you're not sure whether a line has been crossed, and you're just waiting for things to get a little bit worse? she breaks off to ask me over Zoom at this point.

I do know that feeling, I tell her. I know it very, very well.

That's what it was like, she says. I just kept thinking that he hadn't crossed a line yet because he was being kind, and because he wasn't aggressive, and because everything seemed so normal to him.

And, she says, I honestly don't know if I could have spoken or got away if I tried. My throat had just… closed up.

I nod again, and she continues.

As Cleo lay there with the man's hands on her breasts, her thoughts were empty, her throat knotted, unable to free a scream lodged there. When he moved his right hand down between her breasts and onto her stomach, her head became emptier still. Then his crawling hands pushed aside the towel and started massaging her inside her underwear, sensually, the same way he had massaged her neck.

I was completely, utterly frozen, she says to me now, five years later.

His hand stayed there for long minutes, for what felt like an eternity. She could feel hot tears prickling behind her eyes, but as far as she knows none of them escaped.

And then, the strangest, strangest thing. The thing she still worries about. The thing that makes her voice soften even further. Lying there, frozen on the massage table, a stranger's dirty hands shoved inside her, Cleo had an orgasm. She only had one thought in that moment: Will my boyfriend ever forgive me for this?

The man smiled a wretched smile and told her to get dressed. She hopped down the stairs as quickly as she could and dived out of the front door of the day spa. She felt completely unanchored, like she might blow away. She needed to sit down.

There's a coffee shop right next to the spa, she tells me.

But I already know this, I think, because I used to go to that same coffee shop and drink tea and eat biscuits after my own massages, prolonging the time I could spend in that relaxed haze.

I don't know why I did that, she tells me now over Zoom. She is stammering. Why did I do that? It seems crazy.

It's not crazy at all, I say in my clearest, most definite voice.

Cleo sat at a window table in the coffee shop and did nothing, thought nothing, for what could have been hours. She didn't understand what had just happened. She was terrified but could still feel the whispers of leftover pleasure in her body. How could that be?

Eventually, she got up from the table, realizing that the massage therapist probably came to this cafe regularly for his afternoon pick-me-up, and walked to her car. It wasn't until she was inside that she started crying. She called her boyfriend and told him what had happened.

I think I was assaulted, she said into the phone, crying.

When she got to the end of the story, her boyfriend said, Wow, that's so bizarre. Let's talk about it later when I meet you at the party. And with that, his voice was gone, and Cleo was alone again.

Next, she called the day spa and left a message on its answering machine, explaining what had happened, and asking for an immediate call-back.

After a few hours of processing the experience, Cleo thought she was ready to go to the party. She arrived at the small house backing on to a busy lane, and tracked down her boyfriend. About an hour later, Cleo realized she couldn't cope, and she asked him if they could go home.

No, he said. I want to stay. I'll just stay at mine tonight and we can talk tomorrow.

For the second time that night, he disappeared, and for the second time that night, she overlooked it. This was a betrayal that fell in line with the one she had experienced earlier that day, and they fed off each other in her mind and convinced her that she didn't deserve anything more from him.

She woke up groggy and soon received a call from the day spa, offering her a free massage to make up for the assault.

When Cleo tells me this part over Zoom, we end up in fits of maniacal laughter. What else could we do?

·   ·   ·

Riley was only twenty when she went to the police. She has just turned twenty-one when we speak. But she doesn't seem it – she is clear, well-spoken, confident, articulate. It's funny how much I find myself admiring the people I speak to for this book. I stare and stare at them on Zoom, think about how brave and clever they are for being able to put their experiences into words. I still shame myself for doing exactly the same thing, but that same act reflected onto them seems, to me, marvellous.

I really, really believed it was my choice.

That is one of the first things Riley says to me when I speak to her in 2020.

I needed it to be my choice, she says next.

Riley grew up in a small town in Australia, near the beach. She went to the comprehensive high school until grade eleven, age sixteen, but found that she had to move because the small school would not let her study music, her first and only love.

Riley is a viola player. She has been all her life. Playing the viola was the biggest part of her life as a teenager, and she couldn't envisage not having a music qualification on her school leaving certificate, because that would mean she wouldn't be able to move away to study the viola at university.

So for her final year, Riley moved to a new high school. It wasn't pleasant. She didn't fit in with the other kids; they were cliquey and exclusive after five years of school together, and she was an outsider.

She was also a very naive sixteen-year-old – she didn't drink or party or take drugs, she told me. She had never even lied to her parents. After school she would go straight home and get her schoolwork done and practise her instrument until bedtime.

Riley was also the only student in her school taking music at a senior level. She spent a lot of time in the music room, always alone or with her music teacher. Because the viola was such a big part of her life and the teacher was the only person who understood this, they became close very quickly.

She had only been at the school for a few weeks when he kissed her for the first time. He was forty-three and had been married for twenty years. She was seventeen and alone. That day was the beginning of a pattern of abuse that would continue for four years.

During her final year at school, Riley and the teacher had an intense relationship. They sneaked around together at school and became closer and closer. At the time, Riley thought of it as an affair. She didn't tell anyone, and neither did he. But the push and pull of the relationship took its toll on her and she was in pain, a heavy weight on her chest all the time. She talked to him about what she was feeling because she couldn't tell anyone else – and she was a teenage girl and needed to express it somehow – but he rarely responded well.

One day, Riley broke down in English class. She didn't know why exactly, or why that day, that morning. But she started crying at her desk and she ran to the toilets and cried for hours. Eventually a teacher found her there and brought her to the office. The principal and leadership team got together to discuss what had happened. Then they sat Riley down and told her that her grades were slipping and that this was unacceptable, that they were concerned. But they didn't ask what she was crying about. This was the first in a long line of ways in which the people and institutions around her would make her feel as though she, and not the abuser, was the problem. As though she – and not he – was the rotten thing that needed to be exorcized.

Riley finished high school and the relationship continued. They would meet up whenever they could and he would chase her whenever she tried to put distance between them. Eventually she tried to end the relationship, to say they should just be friends.

One day not long after, she got a call from him. He was elated, saying he had started seeing someone new. Her stomach twisted. He told her he was dating one of the teachers at her school. She pictured the woman's face. Then he told her that they had been sneaking around and hooking up in all the dark, shady parts of the school where he had taken her, and the knot in her stomach intensified. It is the first time she remembers thinking: This is a pattern of his.

She insisted that she really just wanted to be friends.

Okay, he said, you're right, let's be friends. Come over for dinner tonight and we can catch up.

Okay, she said, hesitant but hopeful.

When she arrived, he immediately started touching her in the same way he had on that first day, in the music room, years earlier. She realized he was using exactly the same progression of intimacy, repeating that first illicit boundary-crossing. Riley wanted him more than she had ever done that night, and it made her think again about patterns, about the kind of sex she had learned to value.

They ended up sleeping together that night, and when they woke in the morning Alex – her teacher – was panicked.

This is cheating, he said, referring to the teacher he was dating at the time. I'm not okay with it, he added, and Riley almost laughed as she thought about his wife and children.

He shut down that morning. The feeling of being pushed away was too much for her, and when she left she vowed it would be the last time she would be close to him. This is a promise to herself that she has kept.

As she was now studying music at university, she tried to focus on her instrument. But music reminded her of him, and she struggled with his absence. Her mental health suffered more and more. She spiralled into depression and anxiety and her university work was deteriorating, and she thought about how her principal had lectured her after that day in English class.

She got a therapist, and he helped a lot, but she knew she couldn't tell him about Alex. She had been a minor when their relationship started, and she knew he would have to report it to police under Australia's mandatory reporting laws.

Riley had started googling things like 'grooming' and 'abuse', but she still couldn't quite square it with what she had experienced. I really needed it to be my choice, she says to me now.

She tried to get on with things, but it got harder and harder to cope. One morning, she snapped. She decided she had to tell someone. She had to place this story outside herself so that she could start to make sense of it.

That morning, Riley had an appointment with her therapist, and she walked into the room feeling nervous and jittery. She started asking questions about his disclosure obligations, saying just enough so that he could tell her what he would be obliged to report but not enough so that he had a clear picture of what was going on. Eventually, she got her answer. He would have to report it, yes, he told her gently.

She told him the story from start to finish. About starting school, about meeting Alex, about the relationship. When she finished, she said: I should tell the police, shouldn't I?

Yes, he said more gently still, and I suggest you do it sooner rather than later.

She nodded and left his office. She went to her lecture that morning, and when she got back to the apartment in central Adelaide where she lived alone, she decided that today was as good a day as any other. She resolved to call the police and ask what the process would involve, just so she could get the ball rolling.

Riley held her breath as the dialling tone drilled into her ear. An officer answered, and Riley asked her a few general questions about making a report about child abuse.

Who was the teacher? the officer said. What is the name of the school?

Riley froze. Do I have to tell you all of this now? she asked.

I just need a few basic details, the woman said. You don't have to make a full statement now.

Riley exhaled. Okay, she said. She whispered the information the woman had asked her, realizing that she had now started a process she could not stop.

After she called the police, Riley decided it was time to tell someone else what had happened to her. She called a friend, and told her everything. Her friend listened on the end of the phone for hours and offered her the sympathy and comfort she needed. To Riley's surprise, she did not force Riley to deal with her own discomfort. She just sat with it, and she listened.

A few days later, Riley was scheduled to make a full statement to the police. She was so aware of herself as she walked through the doors of the station. At home that morning, she had spent hours wondering what a person who is telling the truth looks like. What does an abuse victim wear? she kept thinking.

Riley sat down in a small room with a male police officer. He asked her straight away if she was comfortable making the report to him.

She was relieved, and she liked him. She said yes. The officer had to fill out paperwork before the statement started, so she sat and watched him, tired and afraid but feeling resolute.

She told the story from start to finish, for only the third time in her life.

He had so many questions for her. How many times a week would you meet up? How many times in total were you intimate with one another?

Panic rose in her chest as she worried that he did not believe her. She did not have all the answers.

But then the officer asked if she had told her parents.

N-no, Riley said, afraid. I decided to tell you first.

Okay, he said softly. There's no need to be scared. Remember that your parents will be angry with him and not with you. You have done nothing wrong.

Riley exhaled for what felt like the first time since she'd walked into the room.

She expected the report to take fifteen minutes. It took two hours. When it was over she called two of her close male friends, and they quickly came and found her. The three of them walked down to the river and sat on the banks and talked late into the evening. She was crying as they sat there, and they tentatively asked her what was wrong. She told them everything. They were sympathetic and kind.

The next day, Riley realized she had left some important things at Alex's house. Now that she had gone to the police, she thought, she needed to get them back. Everything needed to end now.

She texted him and they met up in town a few days later. He had no idea she had reported him. He was snide and arrogant and rude, as he could be sometimes. Even though he didn't know the details, he could already sense on this day that he was being shut out. It was the last time they would ever see each other outside of a courtroom.

Riley had made her report at a police station in the nearest big city, far from the country town where she went to school. So the officers completed the report and the paperwork and then referred the case to a detective in the town where Riley grew up. The detective called Riley to check in as soon as she was placed on the case. She was sensitive and thorough and kind. She asked questions and checked in often, and referred her to the police's victim support services. She told Riley that she had notified the school of the complaint.

Alex was arrested and formally charged. The school sent out a letter about the arrest. It read: In order to protect the victim's privacy, we ask that you refrain from sharing this news on social media. She scoffed. When I speak to Riley about this in 2020, she tells me it was straight out of the private school sex scandal textbook.

That wasn't for me, she says to me, laughing. That was for them. They never asked me what I wanted.

· · ·

Victoria calls me a second time from her home in coastal Australia on a Saturday night, after dinner and drinks with her close female friends. We have scheduled our interview for around the time she usually gets home, 9 p.m. Her friends had drinks, but she did not. She is sober, she tells me.

We chat easily, like we are already friends. Her voice is self-assured and soothing. I can tell she is older than me, but not by much. She continues her story with a confidence that settles and comforts me.

Victoria says that she eventually recovered, as much as she ever could, from the rape and the failed prosecution. But the scars of it lived on in her body, alongside the ghosts of self-hatred that had taken up residence there years and years earlier.

And from them, something else grew. Victoria found herself drawn to a man who she knew did not treat her properly but who she couldn't seem to stay away from.

They met in Melbourne but he was from Ghana, just like her father. Her isolation and self-hatred in the wake of her rape led her to accept his emotionally abusive behaviour without questioning it, she tells me, and soon he was making her feel worse and worse about herself. About a year into their relationship, Victoria found herself pregnant and her partner pushed her to get a termination. She tells me she still doesn't know how severely this procedure impacted her. She knows it left a wound, and she suspects the depth of it is yet to reveal itself.

She became pregnant again the following year, and the couple had a son. She wanted so badly for the relationship to get better, but it did not. After a period of living and raising their son in Ghana, her partner became more and more abusive, and eventually left them. Victoria moved with her son back to Australia, where she is still living when I speak to her.

.   .   .

After the police arrested Riley's teacher, they called her and told her they needed an addendum statement from her. She sat across a table from an officer and identified naked photos of her that police had found in Alex's possession. Yes, that's me, yes, I'm sure, she said, over and over again.

Riley was desperately trying to keep on top of her university work while the police were collecting evidence for the trial, but it was always on her mind. She thought about them digging into his past, about how she had to verify the naked photos of herself they had found on his phone. Will he get convicted? she wondered, again and again, every time she tried to practise her viola or study for her music exams.

The first pretrial court date was scheduled for a Monday in May. When the detective called to tell her, her heart leaped up into her throat and she froze. Every step of this process had been so overwhelming, had so completely engulfed her in anxiety, that she could never think one step ahead, could never turn her mind to what was coming next.

When news of the first court date arrived, Riley realized that she hadn't yet thought about the actual, formal, court part of the process, with lawyers and judges and wigs and a jury. She felt hot and cold at the thought of it. How would she cope with that scenario?

As these thoughts were spinning through her head, the detective told Riley that she did not have to be present at the first hearing, it was mostly procedural, and her presence wouldn't be required.

Thank god, Riley breathed. Then, after a beat: Will he be there?

Yes, the detective said kindly, yes, he will be there.

Okay, Riley said.

That night, as she thought about the idea of him sitting in a courtroom, on trial, her relief at not having to be present started to vanish. Even without having to go, how would she get through that day? How would the anxiety not overwhelm her? How would she fight the urge she had every single day to call him and promise she would take it all back, that she didn't mean it, that she'd keep his secret for him forever? How could she fight the urge to show up at the hearing and shout I OBJECT, as though at a wedding, and force the police to withdraw the charges?

A few days later, Riley was leafing through the programme of a writers' festival in the city she now lived in. As she looked through the booklet, she started to get excited about all the thing she could attend. Then, something stood out to her.

On a Monday in early March, a writer called Bri Lee was giving a talk about surviving sexual abuse. Lee's first book, an incredibly powerful memoir called *Eggshell Skull*, tells the true story of Lee's own struggle against childhood sexual abuse and, remarkably, her decision years later to take on her abuser in court, a case which she won.

The ninth of March: that was the same day as Alex's first hearing. Riley smiled to herself. If there was ever a sign from the universe, this was it.

Reading *Eggshell Skull* had changed her, had lifted her up and given her strength. Lee's story of bravery and power was what had inspired her to disclose her own abuse. The fact that this woman, someone who had meant so much to her, was speaking about the topic on the same day that Alex would appear before a judge for the first time, couldn't be a coincidence.

Now, Riley knew how she was going to get through that terrible day. She would go to university in the morning, buoyed all day by the knowledge that by 5 p.m. she would be sitting under an outdoor tent at the beautiful writers' festival, listening to Bri speak, gaining strength and power from her with every word, every breath.

When Riley arrived at the festival that day, she knew she had made the right decision. She felt proud and powerful, and listening to Bri made her feel sure she had made the right decision.

Riley didn't know me or my writing, but I was onstage with Bri that day. The event was about her abuse memoir as well as my own, and we talked about recovery and disclosure and speaking up. I admire Bri so much, and it was wonderful to get to meet her and do the event with her that day. After the event Riley bought and read my book, which is how we ended up in touch, and how her story ended up on these pages.

When she tells me this, I tear up instantly and uncontrollably. To think that our words that day gave her strength while Alex was brought before the justice system was an unparalleled feeling of joy and awe. I had spent a full year hating the book that I had written, hated that I had drawn so much attention to myself, hated that I had displayed so much repulsive weakness. The first time I didn't feel this self-loathing was sitting on that stage with Bri. Here was someone who had done the same thing as me, and as I listened to her words I began to feel an admiration for her that I couldn't translate to myself. The second time was on my Zoom call with Riley. Hearing that my work had done for her what Bri's had done for me, I felt proud for the first time of what I had made.

All of a sudden, a thought hit me.

Did we meet that day? I asked her. I was internally panicking as I remembered the long line of people whose books I had signed, but also the state of extreme distress I had been in at the time, my mind unravelling after having just exposed myself to an audience for the first time in my life. That event, and the moments after it, are mostly blank. I was completely terrified and in an internal shame spiral. So I couldn't remember if I had met her or not.

I explain this to her, and she smiles and says, No, don't worry, we didn't meet. I exhale.

After a pause she says, I was in line to get you to sign my book when my phone rang. It was my aunt, who had attended the hearing on my behalf so that she could tell me the little things I didn't feel like I could ask the detectives: What was he wearing? Did he bring anyone with him? His new girlfriend? His *parents*?

How did he seem? Riley asked over the phone.

Arrogant at first, her aunt said. But then when the hearing was over and his lawyer was speaking to opposing counsel and he was alone at the defence table for a moment, just for that moment, he looked afraid.

He looked afraid, Riley repeated to herself.

To me, over Zoom, she says: And it was all worth it. Just for that one moment, I had the power to make him feel afraid. That moment when my aunt said that over the phone was the best I've felt since I met him.

I think about the fact that Riley was standing on the grass only a few feet away from me when she took that call, when she felt that power. We had never met, but we were already so connected. A thing like that.

It is the school that Riley feels most let down by, she tells me. I can see the resignation in her eyes as she tells me about how, years later when she was herself qualifying to be a music teacher in a high school, she had to take a module about how to recognize children who are being abused or groomed by teachers.

They should have known, she says to me now, over Zoom. All the signs were there. They should have known.

I nod and nod.

And I know I never said anything, but still, she trails off, and I cut in.

But it's not our job to know what's going on, I say. It's theirs. Abuse only works if we ourselves have been led to feel unsure about our own boundaries, about what we deserve. Groomed children cannot stand up for themselves. Adults have to do it for us. We cannot see what is happening to us, but they can, if they know where to look.

She nods.

Have you heard about the fly in the bottle? I ask, and she shakes her head.

I tell her the story. Riley nods and blinks back tears.

It wasn't our job to see the bottle, I say. It's impossible. Adults can see the bottle if they are looking for it, and they should have intervened. Someone should have intervened to protect you. Nothing is your fault.

· · ·

Cleo calmly explained to the manager that she would not be returning to the spa for another massage as long as she lived, free or otherwise. She asked about the perpetrator's punishment.

The manager said he was a contractor, so it was very difficult to discipline him. She asked Cleo if there was anything else she could do, and Cleo said no and hung up the phone, despondent and exhausted.

That afternoon she went to her boyfriend's house. He still lived with his parents, and she felt so uncomfortable in their presence, in this foreign home, when all she wanted to do was break down.

Instead, she did the only thing she knew she was good at. She started building her case as though she were a lawyer.

She wrote down every detail she could remember about that afternoon. She found the exact times of each of the distressed phone calls she had made and who they were to, all logged on her iPhone as evidence. She had already showered but she found her dirty clothes from the day before and shoved them into her bag. With a meticulous statement in hand, she went to the local police station.

The police agreed to take a full statement from her the next morning at 9 a.m. It would be the first time she had taken even an hour off work in her new job.

The statement was gruelling and took most of the morning. Afterwards, Cleo walked back into her small office, but when the solicitor who sat next to her tried to say hello her throat closed up and tears came, so she simply placed a printed copy of her statement on her desk to explain her absence, and left.

The man was not arrested for another nine months. As those days wore on, Cleo began to recall something he had done in their first massage session, the one where nothing had gone wrong. Afterwards, citing the extreme tension in her back, he handed her a business card with his mobile number on it. He told her he sometimes did treatments from home for his regular customers.

Was this his regular tactic? she thought. Making sure customers always came to him, then moving the treatments to his home, where he could go further than he had with her? The thought haunted her endlessly during those months before he was arrested.

Everyone at work knew about the assault, and Cleo's colleague at the adjacent desk started asking her incessant questions about how it was going. He kept saying she would surely lose. I'm a defence lawyer, he would say, and I know for sure that that orgasm will bring down the whole case. When she tells me this over Zoom, I wonder why on earth her boss did not protect her from this.

A few weeks later, her team received another child sex abuse case. It wasn't a strong case, so her colleague at the next table immediately said he didn't want to do it. Cleo was desperate for a distraction and knew that her boss would be expecting her to pick up any slack, so she volunteered. But she didn't anticipate how the case would affect her.

Cleo knew something bad had happened. She knew she had been assaulted. She knew she felt violated. By telling her friends, her boyfriend and the police, she had convinced herself that she had exorcized the ghost of it. But she hadn't.

As part of its programme for victims of crime, the police had offered Cleo free, state-funded counselling to help her recover. Her counsellor didn't take her experience particularly seriously, and she didn't feel it was helping. Cleo asked the police to switch, but they said no. It would be over a year before Cleo got a proper diagnosis of post-traumatic stress disorder. In the months immediately after the assault, she was angry and irritable, crying in toilets in courthouses, unable to sleep, waking in the early hours with nightmares, but was convinced she had not been affected by what happened that day.

While representing a perpetrator in the child sex abuse case, Cleo started unravelling. The evidence she had to sit through was graphic and kept giving her flashbacks to feeling frozen and afraid in the room with the purple walls and low-humming classical music. She kept breaking down at work, but neither her boss nor her colleagues registered that a victim of sexual assault should not be forced to run a sexual assault case on her own, or at all.

After a few months of counselling, her state-funded therapist tried to discharge her, saying she had 'graduated'.

Most victims of single-incident trauma recover within two months or so, so there's no way you should still be having symptoms, the counsellor said, and sent Cleo on her way.

When Cleo gets to this part of the story, it is my turn to find words frozen in my throat. I cannot believe the extent of his grand, insulting failure. I am so angry at this counsellor that I want to scream, I want to yell and throw things. I blink back tears.

When I was raped, no one helped me because no one knew. No one knew because I was so afraid that if I told anyone, they would refuse to help me. In the end, it was my therapists who saved my life. It was only because I knew I could trust them to listen that I ever opened up about my abuse. They were my last line of defence. They so often are. And for Cleo, they were just another weapon in the arsenal of those who wish to convince us that our persistent pain is not real.

Cleo is speaking again now, and she can sense my anger and sadness.

It just feels so unfair, she says. I am one of the lucky ones. I tell myself every single day that I should have recovered from this more quickly, I don't need a professional shaming me for exactly the same reasons.

It is so unfair, I say. So often, in these interviews, I find that's all I am able to say, and it's not nearly enough.

Most people would have given up after that. I certainly would have. But Cleo didn't. She called up the day spa, remembering they had offered to help in any way they could, and asked if she could have the refund to put towards therapy, but they refused. She pushed the state and the police again and again until they gave her a new therapist.

Then a scandal exploded in Australian politics. A high-profile news show aired an investigation into torture and abuse being inflicted on Indigenous children in Australian prisons. The story was truly, gut-wrenchingly horrifying. It electrified the country. Everyone was outraged.

A few days later, Cleo's boss asked her if she would move to the city where the case was located and run their entire operation from there, managing the high-profile case from start to finish. She was overwhelmed and still not sleeping but she knew it was the case of a lifetime, so she said yes.

She moved cities, and she and her boyfriend agreed that he would come to visit a month later. They hadn't spoken much about the assault or the police since the day after it had happened, so she rarely told him how much she was struggling. He seemed not to notice that she cried most nights as she lay next to him.

The move was hard and the case was more difficult than she had ever imagined. The young man who was the public face of the case was her main client, and she drove to visit him in prison daily. When he spoke about trauma and fear, she found herself saying: I think I know a tiny bit about what that's like. The two got on incredibly well, and he trusted her.

As she became more and more overwhelmed, she contacted the organization that arranges counselling for victims of crime to schedule some extra sessions. But they informed her that a victim can only receive support in the state in which the crime was committed, and as Cleo had moved states, she was no longer entitled to anything.

Cleo hung up, wanting to scream at the officer that surely she was not the first person to desperately want to move thousands of miles away after being assaulted.

Cleo's boyfriend came to Darwin and the two went out to a very expensive restaurant to celebrate an anniversary. The next morning, as he left for the airport, he broke up with her.

In all the hours that she speaks, Cleo never mentions whether or not her attacker was convicted. I'm not sure if she is aware that she has left this out, but I want to let it stand on its own, this absence. If it is not important to her, then it is not important to me. Like I said, this book isn't about him.

CHAPTER TEN

Rape is both unbearably traumatic and something we are expected to bear with alarming regularity. It is very confusing to know in your body that something is dangerous but be told again and again, in so many different ways, that it is just a standard occupational hazard. It seems that this cruel combination of something being both life-altering and everyday leads us to never be quite sure which narrative is true and which is not. We have come to only be able to understand our sexual assaults when they are refracted off a different surface.

I could only understand my rape when I got sick ten years later and could see my body breaking down. I have friends who have told me they could only understand their own assaults when they heard a story about someone else experiencing the same thing. Pema could only understand her rape when it was written about in an academic journal. In this chapter, Charlie questions her rape because of a smiley face on a form.

I question my own assault still. I sit across the room from my therapist and say: Was it real? Did it happen? How can I be sure? How can I trust myself if no one else trusts me?

Life after rape is a paradox. The tug between one life and another, that liminal space. Confusion about the distinction between sex and violence, care and abuse, reality and fiction. The author Rosie Price said that in writing *What Red Was*, her novel about surviving sexual assault, she focused on two words: *Burial / resurfacing*.

I feel like that captures it perfectly.

Narratives about rape being uncommon clash with our experience of it being always just around the corner. Light-hearted jokes about consent are at odds with our bone-deep knowledge that rape is life-threatening. Narratives about rape only being committed by monsters stand in stark contrast to our experiences with partners, family members and friends. The constant recalibration of a worldview, the struggle between the world we live in as survivors and the one those of us on the outside of this experience would have us believe, is real.

Inside us there is an endless tug between burial and resurfacing, burial again, resurfacing, not knowing if it will ever stop.

In this memory, it is 2 a.m. and I am lying on my side on the landing outside my flat. I have just fallen down a flight of stairs, tumbled out of my front door, which I didn't realize I'd left on the latch, and have landed hard against the wooden floor at the bottom.

I am surrounded by chipped paint and old receipts that have fallen out of my messy handbag at various points over the last year as I have rifled through it to find my keys. The landing is dark and stuffy.

I have a duvet pulled tight around me, and I held it close to me as I tumbled, so I am not too badly bruised. But I have pulled a muscle in my back and I find myself unable to move for several minutes. So I lie there, naked under the duvet, which is pure white except for the bloodstains it is now splashed with. I am bleeding but I don't know it yet, so the blood is silently leaking onto the white fabric like a poorly kept secret, like proof that I will never be as clean as I pretend to be.

I am not bleeding because I was raped, although I have been raped before.

The man I am dating is asleep upstairs in my flat. He has no idea that I am in trouble. He has no idea that I am lying at the bottom of the stairs, and he never will. It seems enormously important that I keep things this way.

Adrienne Rich says in her book *Women and Honor: Some Notes on Lying*, that women are forced so often to lie with their bodies, and about their bodies, through their bodies, that they end up losing touch with themselves. They deprive themselves of a part of their own lives. But, she writes, 'The unconscious wants truth, as the body does.'

And they will find this truth. Eventually the body and the unconscious mind will push you down the stairs and leave you naked on the landing, hurting, bleeding, unable to maintain the lie.

My date and I had a very nice evening together. I was in pain that night, so I knew that sex would be unbearably painful. I knew my date would understand why I couldn't, and I resolved to abstain.

But as the last of the evening light faded – it was summer in London, and the last light lingered in the sky until almost 11 p.m. – I started getting an uneasy, fluttering feeling, like there were caged birds beating their wings in my chest. I felt like he was losing interest, like I'd lost his attention. I became convinced that he had realized what I had always known: that I am a rotten thing who does not deserve to be loved. That my wretchedness is a poison that will infect anyone who comes too close. My muscles felt an urge to run – not away from him, but towards him. I needed him not to leave.

When this happens, something catches fire inside of me. I need, more than anything, for this person to come to me. To love me even though I am a girl made of poison. To love me even though I am desperately afraid to be loved. That feeling of total unworthiness is typical of abuse survivors, but I did not know this yet.

When I need to be sure of a bond, I use physical intimacy as my glue. I have always been taught to believe that it's the only thing that works.

While we were lying there that night, I felt so scared I could hardly breathe. He fell asleep immediately and I lay there next to him, clutching my stomach, frozen. I left the bedroom on tiptoe, taking the duvet with me, and sat at the top of my stairs thinking about what I could do, where I could go. I was in a state of total panic. I kept having flashbacks to the sex we had just had, how it had made me feel so worthless, how there was nothing in the world that made me hate myself more than using sex to create intimacy. So why had I done it?

All of a sudden my desperation to get away became much stronger. I needed to run. Without thinking about where I would go, I stood up quickly and stepped towards the staircase and I fell and tumbled down, and the next thing I knew I was lying naked at the bottom of the stairs.

Nora Salem says in 'The Life Ruiner', her own essay about abuse:

> Perhaps the most horrifying thing about non-consensual sex is that, in an instant, it erases you. Your own desires, your safety and well-being, your ownership of a body that may very well be the only thing you felt sure you owned.

I have never had an intimate heterosexual experience that did not make me want to disappear.

Before I was raped in 2007, I had never had sex. I had never engaged in any kind of intimacy, not really. His was the first and only sexual script I have ever known. I say first and only because this is how sexual abuse works – it imprints itself on us and we, in turn, imprint it upon everything that comes near us. The assault lasted about twenty minutes, but fragments of it will last a lifetime.

For ten years, every sexual experience I had was painful and terrifying. I had not spoken about the rape to anyone, and I hadn't even acknowledged it to myself, so I didn't make the connection between the attack and my fear of intimacy. I thought it was normal. And girls are taught never to talk about sex in any detail, so there were no opportunities to correct this assumption. I forced myself to engage in sex with men because the world taught me to believe that it was a prerequisite for intimacy and care. Physical closeness terrified me, but I wanted emotional support more than anything. I wanted it so desperately it felt like sometimes the need would swallow me up, propel me into a dark, dank place where no love could ever reach me.

I wanted so badly to be cared for. I wanted so badly to be seen. Because I am human, but also because I was suffering. I was trying to face a world that had all of a sudden become threatening and fragile and wretched. I was trying to understand how it could be that I had ever felt safe, that I had ever felt comfortable. I was trying to connect with the person I was before the attack, but she was far away, and so was everybody else.

Everywhere I looked I saw romantic love – and sexual intimacy – reflected back at me. That was the only path to a meaningful connection with another person, and I wanted that connection so badly I would do anything for it. Even the thing that frightened me the most. Even the thing I was least able to bear.

Sexual acts became a performance. Something I had to tolerate so that I could be entitled to the friendship and support that came with it. Everything about my intimate life was an act. I learned from films and TV what kind of sounds I should make, how women's faces are supposed to look when they are enjoying physical touch.

My lived experience of these things was built on a memory of sharp pain, blurred vision, blackout, a Swiss army knife plunged into trembling skin. I had no idea what sexual pleasure felt like, and I didn't trust myself to imagine it, so I performed. I found ways to manoeuvre myself so the person I was sleeping with couldn't see my face, so that just for a minute I could let the pain show. I could squeeze my eyes shut and cry without breaking the fourth wall. Without fracturing the fantasy.

One of the lesser-known after-effects of trauma is that it makes the survivor hyper-vigilant and hyper-attuned to everything around themselves. Their senses become primed to detect danger. They pick up on signals invisible to others: every slight adjustment in body language, every double take, every stolen glance gets catalogued into a database in the mind that is always weighing whether or not it is time to run.

This made me particularly good at performing intimacy. I was so attuned to people that I could figure out what they wanted from me, and I could become that person, like magic. The more I worked on my performance, the more comfortable I felt. The act was something I hid behind. I needed it to be a sexual identity so real that there was nothing left that might prompt a partner to question my past.

This is how I led romantic relationships for ten years.

I fell in love and out of it, but I was never wholly honest about myself. The people who got closest to me physically were the people who knew me the least, the people I lied to the most.

I found ways in my everyday life to hide the fact that I hated being touched, that I couldn't stand physical proximity. I learned to hide my discomfort when friends held my hand or patted my shoulder. I learned how to exit a conversation without ever having to hug anyone, making sure to leave only when people were positioned in such a way that getting up to embrace me would be a hassle.

I learned to talk about enjoying sex too, reading scripts from the girls I knew and the women in the novels I devoured. I learned what people wanted to hear. I became good at lying.

'There is a danger run by all powerless people,' Adrienne Rich says, 'that we forget we are lying, or that lying becomes a weapon we carry over into relationships with people who do not have power over us.'

I came so close to forgetting that I was lying. I couldn't acknowledge the truth because the grief of it was too heavy. Nora Salem asks: 'Am I ruined, after all? Answering that would require me to imagine a world in which this never happened to me. What would I look like? Act like? How would I love?'

I couldn't bear the thought.

The first time I went to see my psychotherapist – the doctor most formative in my recovery – we were sitting in a very small room with two big chairs and barely any space between them. He said I looked uncomfortable, and asked if I was okay.

Without thinking, I stammered, I don't like sitting this close to you.

He said, Do you feel that way about most people, or just men?

Mostly men, I said, thinking about it properly for the first time.
Why do you think that is? he asked.

Before I knew what was happening, I was telling him the story of my rape. It was the first time I had properly spoken about it aloud.

After this first disclosure, I started seeing a sex therapist who specialized in the after-effects of trauma. She taught me how to stop myself from dissociating every time I was touched. She was the first person to teach me that sex was supposed to be enjoyable, and not something I had to trade for something else. Sex wasn't just an offering, a blood sacrifice.

I have been working with two sex therapists for a year now, and each week they teach me something new about myself. I am still scared of physical closeness, but I am also full of wonder – there's a whole world out there, it turns out, that I've never been able to see. A whole side of my personality that was taken in the night and never given back.

My therapist explains to me that our intimate sexual side is deeply connected to creativity and empathy – two of the things I value most. I feel hot with anger as I realize that the man in the empty toilet stall has taken these things from me, taken sides of myself I cherish so much. But as the anger passes, it is replaced by something like excitement. I know that I can't undo what happened to that girl, but I can approach her with curiosity. I can say: I know you have suffered beyond measure, and I want to understand who you have become. What do you look like? Act like? How do you love? What do you wish to create?

That night when I found myself lying on my side on the landing outside my flat forced me to accept that of all of the elements of my recovery – the terror, the nightmares, the operations, the pain, the loneliness – intimacy is the hardest.

Maybe you cannot build love from a crime scene. Maybe this is one thing my attacker took from me that I will never recover. I'm not even sure if I want to. Perhaps it's better not to know the extent of what you have lost.

What I have been able to do is accept the truth of my intimate self. I know now that she is bloodied and broken, and perhaps damaged beyond repair. But I am trying, and will keep trying, because whoever was buried under the weight of abuse is worth fighting for.

I've stopped lying with my body as a way of extracting love from others. I have realized that I can be honest about what I've lost, about what I cannot bear, to those I am close to, and if they know – as I now do – that this is not my fault, then they will stay and help me wrestle with the pain.

Trying to navigate love and accept affection without the deceit I spent so many years perfecting is singularly terrifying, because it means I risk having the one thing I fear most confirmed: that my body, mauled by a stranger in the night, makes me difficult to love. But that's a risk I have to take, because it's the only way to open myself up to true connection. It's the only way I will ever love and be loved in the way that I want to be. The truth is that I am a desperate, hopeless romantic. I want to be giddy and smitten and besotted and understood and cared for, no matter how hard it is to get there. If I give up on that kind of love, if I keep lying, then I will let my attacker take something from me that is more important than my creativity, or my safety, or even my body. I cannot let him take the part of me that believes in love.

As I watch people walk away when it gets too hard, as I find myself defeated and wanting to return to my performed self, I think of Adrienne Rich in *On Lies, Secrets, and Silence*: 'When a woman tells the truth she creates the possibility of more truth around her.'

Even if insisting on being honest about my suffering makes me difficult to love, it's worth it, because the act of telling the truth is a revolution. An act of kindness that I finally know I deserve; an act of kindness that might also open up the possibility of love for others; an invisible gesture that, if repeated, might just balance out the cruelty this world contains.

I think of the psychoanalyst Donald Winnicott's observation in

Maturational Processes and the Facilitating Environment: 'It is a joy to be hidden but disaster not to be found.'

. . .

One of Jules' friends, Matt, visited them in Brussels from Leeds. Matt was kind and gentle, and the friends were close. But the relationship had also been ambiguous at times. When Matt and Jules first met, they had a semi-flirtatious relationship, at least on his side. Since then they had settled into a nice platonic friendship, but Jules wanted to clarify the terms of the holiday anyway.

I would love to hang out, but we don't have a spare bedroom. So you'll have to sleep on the couch, they told Matt on the phone one night.

That's fine! he chirped.

When Matt arrived, the friends went out on the town together and Jules introduced him to their friends and their favourite bars. It was nice, seeing Brussels through the eyes of a visitor, getting to show it off. The two of them drank and danced, and Jules was enjoying themself until they got home.

Jules pulled out clean linen from the cupboard and made up the sofa carefully, making sure Matt was comfortable. Then Jules said goodnight and went into their bedroom, closing the door behind them.

Sometime in the night, Jules was jolted awake by their creaky bedroom door opening. Matt shuffled towards Jules and climbed into bed next to them, murmuring something sleepily. Jules felt uncomfortable, but they were also underneath a heavy fog of sleep and dreams, so they stayed still, facing the wall, hoping he would just fall asleep next to them.

But instead, Matt's arms clawed at Jules. His fingers, cold from the winter night and the cold flat, gripped onto Jules' waist, less sleepily than his night-time shuffle had indicated. He was wide awake.

Jules murmured something and pushed Matt's hands off them, but he grabbed on again, tighter this time. It had been a very long time since Jules had slept with a man, and his body next to theirs felt painfully large and angular. Matt put his right hand into their underwear, and they froze. Then Matt pulled their underwear down and pushed himself inside them, and Jules waited for it to be over.

After the rape, Jules got sicker and sicker, and their mental health started deteriorating even further. They found themself afraid of shadows.

Hearing this part of Jules' story makes me think of Farhana, and every story I have ever heard about women and non-binary people being violated by people we trust, or believing ourselves to be safe when we are not. The line between safety and danger is such a thin one if you live in a girl or a girl-adjacent body.

When I speak to Jules, the world is in lockdown. They have been stuck inside in their Brussels apartment for months. They tell me they are really, really struggling to adapt to these new conditions. They say they think it is causing a flare-up of their symptoms of post traumatic stress syndrome, which have been diagnosed and then have worsened since the rape and their Hashimoto's diagnosis.

Without my usual journalistic restraint, I spring into speech. Me too, I say. I have been thinking so much about how lockdown exacerbates symptoms of trauma, and how those of us with a history of trauma are finding it so much more difficult than others, I add.

Jules nods over Zoom.

I continue: I think it's because the symptoms of post-traumatic stress are so deeply connected to trying to make sense out of chaos and trying to control a terrifying situation. And now all of a sudden we have been thrown into another terrifying situation over which we have no control.

Yes, exactly. Jules nods again.

It's like all my instincts of self-punishment and self-control have been reinvigorated since the world changed overnight, I say, and explain to them that my own eating disorder has returned and that I have lost three kilos in a month.

On the plus side, Jules tells me, they have been using lockdown to explain to their friends that they want to go by the 'they' pronoun from now on, and they are proud of themself for that. They have also spent time writing and editing their poetry, which has made them feel calm again. Also, they say, I learned how to knit. It's so helpful.

I have always wanted to learn to knit! I exclaim, as Jules shows me the scarf they are working on.

Let's arrange another Zoom call and I'll teach you, they say, and I can tell that they mean it, and I nod.

.   .   .

Charlie tells me she has always felt uncomfortable in her body, even before her assault, because she is overweight and has always felt ashamed of that fact. She finds it difficult to connect with the sexual side of her identity because the kind of body she has is never woven into sexual narratives.

Charlie felt at home with her sexuality for the first time when she discovered her local BDSM community and started meeting up with men for casual, BDSM-oriented sex. BDSM is a type of sexual practice, often involving role play, that comprises bondage and discipline, dominance and submission, sadism and masochism. The community was – she thought – inclusive and open and kind, and it made her feel comfortable with her desires and with herself.

One day, she started chatting to a man on the website she primarily used for BDSM dates. The man was friendly and talkative, a single high school teacher who seemed to be on the same page as her. They agreed to meet for a date at a pub near the boarding school where Charlie teaches and lives.

Before the pair met up, the man sent her a list via email of all the things he wanted to try with her, and asked her to indicate whether she would be up for them or not. Charlie was taken aback because the list was so long and had all sorts of wild things on it. But she supposed the list represented a form of active consent, so she filled it in and sent it back.

There was one box that she hesitated over. It read 'consensual non-consent'. This, she tells me, is basically 'rape play', where two consenting partners feign non-consensual sex. Charlie was nervous about her answer, because she had never tried it before and felt instantly pressured. She wrote: *I have never tried this but I might consider it for the right person.*

She put the paper down, picked it up again. She decided to add a smiley face at the end of the sentence, just to lighten the mood.

Now it read: *I have never tried this but I might consider it for the right person* ☺

On their first date, Charlie knew instantly that she was attracted to the man. Soon after he sat down, he pulled a small vibrator out of his pocket and asked her to put it inside her for the date. The vibrator came with a remote-controlled device, which he would have in his hands while they chatted so he could control what the little machine was doing inside her.

Charlie felt uncomfortable about this, but he seemed insistent, and something made her go along with it. She spent the whole evening frantically wondering whether those sitting near her could hear the vibrations or feel them along the shared bench. She was anxious, and she drank beer quickly to try and relieve the feeling.

Overall, though, Charlie figured she was enjoying the date. It wasn't the worst one she'd ever been on. But she drank quickly, and she doesn't remember much about them deciding to go back to her apartment. But she knows that they got there and had sex, which was fine, if not amazing. But when he was finished, the man got up, got dressed in a matter of minutes and just... left.

She felt a knot in her stomach as he left, one that grew and grew in the moments afterwards as she stared at her bedroom wall. She felt unanchored and abandoned.

Charlie starts to explain this feeling to me, but I know it instinctively.

I have felt it so many times. That feeling of being left alone when you are at your most vulnerable, having exposed the most frightening part of yourself only to be left alone with your thoughts. For me, that feeling can be almost unbearable. It sickens me.

But, Charlie is explaining to me over Zoom, this feeling is even more heightened when you are involved with the BDSM community. The kind of sex you have, and enjoy having, is even more exposing than what I have experienced – you have to make yourself so vulnerable to the other person in this world. Charlie explains to me that there is an unspoken agreement, particularly on the first intimate encounter with a particular person, that both parties will support each other afterwards and make sure they feel okay with what has happened.

BDSM often involves role playing, Charlie says to me, and it's so important for someone to support you while you are coming out of that role. When someone wrenches themselves away like that, without warning, people so often – especially women – are left feeling ashamed and afraid of the role they have played, without anyone to take their hand and tell them their desires are valid and real.

I feel so strongly for Charlie when she tells me this. I can't imagine the hurt she would have felt in that moment.

Continuing her story, Charlie tells me that she messaged the man and explained that she did not want to see him again, but he refused to take no for an answer. He kept messaging her, again and again. He called and called. She screened his calls and his messages, but he kept going.

After a few weeks of this, Charlie started to get quite worried. She couldn't stop thinking about the fact that he knew where she lived, knew her address, knew which school she worked at. She kept thinking about the vibrator he had asked her to put inside herself, and about that checklist and all the things he wanted to do with her, and what had bordered on uncomfortable before was starting to feel menacing.

She asked the receptionists at her school's front desk to look out for him, and gave them a detailed description and asked them to alert her if he came on school property. She continued to ignore his calls.

One day, the man texted Charlie, begging for her to hear him out. He just wanted to see her for a quick drink, he said, and then he would stop texting. He stirred something in her, something like guilt, so she agreed.

They met at the pub and he started to explain that he was sorry he had been insensitive and left so quickly the last time, and that he had been thinking about her a lot, and she was flattered. They talked and talked and she started to feel comfortable again, started to question whether her instincts about him were to be trusted.

She doesn't remember inviting him home with her, but she must have, she says to me over Zoom, because that's where they ended up. They started kissing. But before she knew it, he had his hands around her throat. He was strangling her, his grip getting tighter and tighter, and she felt herself losing her breath. She tried to tell him to stop, but she couldn't speak, she could only gasp.

Everything went black.

.   .   .

I cannot write about what it means to live in a female body without writing about what it means to die in a female body. Charlie's story sends me back into another memory, one I haven't revisited since it happened.

In this memory, I am sitting in a bedroom in my north London flat. It has been a few months since I moved here and I have not made any friends. I am so lonely. I spend all of my time in this room, trying to write a memoir about recovery but falling further into despair. I have a routine that involves only waking up late and feeling hazy, trying to write for the afternoon but giving up around 4 p.m. and having my first glass of wine for the evening.

Once safely in my room, I drink and try and forget about writing, and about rape, and about London. To do this, I scroll endlessly through profiles on dating apps and try and start virtual conversations to fill the void.

I am on Tinder, Bumble and Hinge. This is how desperate I am.

I spend hours and hours curating my profile. This is actually a good thing, because I have hours and hours to kill while avoiding writing *I Choose Elena*. So here I am, scrolling through photos of myself and trying to choose which ones will best capture who I think I am trying to be. I choose photos of me with books in my hand to try and establish a strong *personal brand*. I'm a writer, I say to myself. I'm a writer. I'm a writer. But I haven't written anything all day; instead I am busy marketing myself as one to an invisible audience of future potential partners.

I have recently cut all of my hair off in a desperate bid to reclaim my life. I have a new fringe and a bob cut. My hair is its natural colour for the first time in about ten years. It is a mild, mousey brown and I have been dyeing it either jet black or peroxide blonde constantly since I was thirteen.

(This was a funny thing about this point in my life; I was in a very strange sort of purgatory. I was performing confidence and embodiment but I was not really living it. I did not realize this at the time, but looking back I realize that I was playing a role I thought I should be ready to live but wasn't.)

I tell myself I like my new, authentic hair as I choose photos for my dating profile, but I am lying to myself. I hate my hair and I hate the face it now fails to conceal in its newly diminished state. On Tinder, I blindly follow the rules that I openly mock when I am speaking with friends. I include one photo that makes me look like a good girl – smart, bookish, innocent, unthreatening. I include one of me on holiday in Italy – carefree, relaxed, but fake-tanned and posing in front of a town square that took me a whole day to choose and force my sister to snap me in front of.

Next I include a photo of me in a swimsuit so I can show off my figure. This is another strange kind of cognitive dissonance. The truth is I hate my body when I see it in a mirror, but somehow I can like it when it is frozen in an image and viewed through the imagined eyes of prospective partners. And yet the real, physical gaze of men or women I am sleeping with terrifies me more than anything, so why does the digital version momentarily soothe me? I have no idea.

Next I need to write my bio. What to say about myself to all the many prospective dates across London? I settle on 'just moved to London, show me around?' with a little rainbow emoji to signal that I am bisexual. I pore over the images of myself, one after the other, until I am satisfied that this is the best I can do. I start swiping furiously, barely looking at the images that flash up before swiping right, desperate to find some validation no matter who or where it comes from. Every time the app tells me 'it's a match!' my heart fills up a little bit more, and I feel slightly less alone. I send each match exactly the same message, a GIF of a bear waving hello.

Next I move on to Bumble. Bumble is supposed to be the most woman-friendly app, because only women are allowed to start conversations. This is intended to stem the tide of unsolicited dick pics, but everyone knows that even men you have spoken to for days or weeks can suddenly turn into the unsolicited dick pic type at any moment. In any case, it doesn't matter, because all it does is heighten my crippling fear of rejection and ensure that I never start a single conversation with a man or woman on this app.

Am I consciously tailoring my Bumble profile to be slightly different to my Tinder one? I am not sure. Probably. It ends up making me look like the kind of girl who would appeal to bankers and architects.

On Hinge, the most recent arrival on the dating app scene, I fret about my answers to the pithy questions and prompts the app gives you. This is supposed to allow us to show off our personality, but in these months I genuinely feel as though I don't have one. Alone in this room, with this book, with no one to witness me, I feel I have disintegrated.

On Hinge, I start speaking to a man called Mark. He tells me he is a musician, and we fire a few nice messages back and forth. I am drunk, and it is a Friday night, and I do not want to stare at the blank pages of my manuscript for a moment longer. So when he asks me if I would like to get a drink, I think: Fuck it.

I say yes. We agree a time and place, but he quickly changes his mind and asks if I will come to his house instead. I ask him where it is and he tells me a neighbourhood, but I am new to London and I don't know where it is.

I look it up on Google Maps and find that it is forty-five minutes north of me by car, only just inside the M25. For a reason which still remains unclear to me, I say yes.

I am full of wine and self-loathing and I want to get out of my head. I tell myself – like I always do – that casual sex will serve as a distraction for the self-hate, a numbing agent. But this is a fantasy. The truth is the opposite – this is just a way of driving the knife in further. This, too, is a form of self-harm.

I sneak out of the house and drunkenly climb into an Uber that takes me far outside London. I have absolutely no idea where I am, and everything looks sinister and unfamiliar. I arrive at the man's house at about 10 p.m. and he comes downstairs to let me in.

He is leering and smells of beer and cigarettes. He looks nothing like he did in his photos. What the hell am I doing here?

I follow him into an apartment covered in trash and half-empty pizza boxes. I am afraid. He asks me to sit down next to him and for some reason I do. He pulls himself on top of me and pulls me into a tight hug. I am underneath him, and he is crushing me.

I say that I need to get up to go to the toilet and, as quickly as I can, I grab my handbag and run out the door. He follows me for a few steps, then falls behind and lets me go. I order another Uber and am back in my bed by midnight, before anyone notices I had left.

The man in the dirty apartment has since found me on Facebook, Instagram and Twitter and sends me messages constantly. I am terrified of him. I still cannot understand how or why I put myself in his path.

.   .   .

From the darkness, things began to swim back into focus. The walls of Charlie's bedroom, the carpet. Sensations came creeping back a few seconds after the images did, as though the physical feelings were crawling slowly up to her brain from her body. After a moment, she registered that he was inside her.

Behind her, the man was raping her. She lay there, waiting for it to be over. He got dressed.

Charlie walked around in a daze for months after her rape. She went to work at the boarding school, came back to her on-campus flat, went to work again. But she felt separated from it all. Even the girls, the ones she was in charge of caring for, the ones she loved so much, felt far away.

One Friday morning, she escorted the girls to their local church. They went to this church once a term, so she was familiar with it, but she wasn't religious herself. The girls filed in and sat through the service, which included a sermon. They listened: the older ones giggled, the younger ones stared up deferentially, and they filed out.

As she walked with the girls, Charlie caught one side of a familiar face, standing in a doorway, facing outside so she could only see part of his profile. As if feeling her gaze, the face turned towards her, and then she was sure. It was her rapist – in a vicar's robes.

Averting her eyes, hoping he wouldn't notice, Charlie turned to a woman near her who worked at the church.

Who is that? she asked the woman.

Oh, that's the vicar of our parish. We adore him. He and his wife and children spend half their lives in this church.

Charlie felt her heart rise into her throat. But at the same moment, she saw that the man had seen her and was walking towards her, so she spun around and stumbled out of the door, down the street, and felt as though she didn't take another breath until she got home.

When I speak to Charlie, she has moved to a new town, to a new house, and a new life. She didn't want to run into the vicar again, or the wife and children he had lied about. She has just moved into her new place when we speak on Zoom. House prices are infinitely more reasonable where she now lives than in some other parts of the UK, and she has a three-bedroom house to herself. We laugh as she tells me how grown-up it feels, at only twenty-nine, to have all this space of her own.

· · ·

Another memory comes to mind, something that happened to me about a month after my interview with Charlie.

I am talking to another boy on Tinder. He works in publishing and he seems interesting, so we decide to meet for a drink.

He is tall and handsome and he seems kind. We talk about books and holidays. At one point he says he likes girls who are 'mysterious' and difficult to figure out. I wonder if this is an intentional dig at the fact that I am writing a memoir at twenty-six. I'm not the girl for you, my friend, I think. I am an open book. Literally.

I am drinking house white wines fast.

I get drunk quickly and my intense feelings of self-loathing rise up in me like waves. As I drink, I get more and more disgusted with myself. I can hear myself slurring and making ridiculous comments.

When he asks me to come home with him, I agree immediately. I do not remember how we get there, or where he lives. We climb two flights of stairs to get to his bedroom and he pulls off my clothes immediately. I am barely conscious. I have had so much wine. He is on top of me with his hands around my neck and he is choking me, hard. I can hardly breathe.

I wait until he is finished and I get up and leave. I get myself home and into bed as quickly as I can.

I have had so much to drink that I fall asleep immediately and do not let myself think about the choking for a few days. When I do, it terrifies me.

For about a week after this night I cannot suppress my feelings of self-hatred. They are alive and angry. I have allowed my body to be violated in a way that it cannot contain.

This is not the first or only time this has happened to me, and I imagine it will not be the last. I am telling you these stories because they are examples of all the many, many ways the female body can be put in danger in everyday life. By others, by ourselves. We are taught that sex is necessary to create connections, but we live in a world – increasingly, with the obsessive use of dating apps – where seeking sex and seeking danger can be indistinguishable from one another. How are we to navigate that?

A 2019 study published in the *Proceedings of the National Academy of Sciences*, 'Disintermediating Your Friends: How Online Dating in the United States Displaces Other Ways of Meeting', by Michael J. Rosenfeld, Reuben J. Thomas and Sonia Hausen, found that heterosexual couples are more likely to meet a romantic partner online than through any other means. So it's easy to see why women increasingly believe that using them is a necessary part of finding love.

Dating has always involved risk. For as long as gendered violence has existed, there has also been a level of danger for women engaging with men. But so many of the safeguards have now been stripped away – the character reviews from friends of friends, the hours of talking in a bar with other friends around before making a decision to be alone with someone. These have all been stripped back by the explosion of dating apps, where we are forced to meet up with men without having any way of knowing if anything they have told us is true, nor if they even are who they say they are.

In December 2018, Grace Millane went on a Tinder date while on her year out in New Zealand. She exchanged messages with the man for a few days before he asked her to meet for a drink. The two had been getting along well, and Grace had texted a friend to say she was excited about the date.

The two had a drink together at a bar he suggested. He seemed nice, and she was enjoying herself. She texted a friend to tell her that they had immediately clicked.

After a few more drinks, the two went home together. But while they were having sex, the man put his hands around Grace's throat and held them there until he suffocated her to death.

After Grace had taken her last breath, the man put her twenty-one-year-old body in a suitcase in the hotel room they were in. He left her there as he went out to buy bleach to clean up the blood that had poured from her nose.

After he came back with the bleach, he left Grace in the hotel room again and went out on another Tinder date. The girl he took for a drink that afternoon had no idea the man had the body of his last Tinder match stuffed in a suitcase in a cheap hotel room, nor that he was living on borrowed time.

After the date, the man took the suitcase with Grace's body inside it downstairs and into his hire car. He drove the body to some nearby woodlands and buried her in a shallow grave, where she was found three days later.

When the man was on trial for her murder, his defence was that Grace had asked for rough sex. That she had consented to being strangled.

The high-profile trial led to questions being asked about this defence, often called the 'rough sex' defence or the 'Fifty Shades' defence, after E.L. James' popular novel about sadomasochistic sex. What the questioners uncovered was alarming: a spike in the number of femicides where this defence was invoked during criminal trials. Underlying this is another disturbing fact: the incidence of this defence has also risen because more men than ever are being accused of killing women during sex.

A man was acquitted in Canada after murdering a sex worker by stabbing her so forcefully in the vagina that her internal organs were punctured, leading her to bleed out while she took shelter in the hotel bathtub as he slept. He woke up to find her dead, checked out and went to work. He said the stabbing was part of the rough sex the woman had consented to, and was acquitted of her murder.

It is legally impossible to consent to your own murder, not in any jurisdiction that I studied for my law degree or read about while researching this book. Yet all over the world, juries are acquitting men who kill women during sex on the basis of an argument that she enjoyed and participated in sexual acts that intimated violence. It feels ridiculous to even write this, but consenting to a game or act that involves pretend violence is not the same as consenting to one's own murder. Those two things can only be equated by juries and courtrooms determined to find a way to blame women for the violence visited upon them.

All of this is to say nothing of the fact that many women only consent to these kinds of acts because they are now so prominent in pornography and, consequently, in the fantasies of men in which women again and again feel pressured to participate. I know what that feels like.

Dating apps and the rise of casual sex have created the perfect storm, where many men feel permitted – without asking first – to act out their fantasies during Tinder dates. This has led to an alarming number of women being strangled by men they have just met.

A recent investigation by the BBC found that more than a third of women under the age of forty in the UK have experienced some degree of unwanted violence during casual sex.

Some of those women will die. Others will become more and more used to it each time it happens; if or when they are eventually harmed or killed, juries will comfort themselves with the knowledge that the woman was okay with it.

I have recently become completely obsessed with true crime, and mostly the kind that depicts violence against women. Why is that? Why did the whole world tune in to *Serial*, and why do I compulsively listen to podcasts about the Golden State Killer, or Ted Bundy, or the man who killed his wife and then set his house on fire with his two small children inside? Is it a way to offset my constant anxiety about being harmed? Like if I look at it directly it won't frighten me as much when it happens?

Here's what else I learned while diving into my obsession with the murder of girls and women. True crime stories purport to shine a light on cruelty but, like every other profitable industry, they do so selectively. Trans people are twice as likely to be victims of crime in the UK than cisgender people, according to data from the Office for National Statistics. Black women in the US are two and a half times more likely to be killed by men than white women, according to a 2015 Violence Policy Center study. But the stories we hear on the podcasts that reopen cold cases are almost exclusively blonde girls who go missing just as they were about to fulfil their endless potential. It is a privilege to have your body looked for.

As I read and write about the women who die from rough sex they 'consented' to, I can't help but think of the last line of Olivia Gatwood's title poem in her new collection, *Life of the Party*, which is all about the epidemic of women dying as a result of male violence. She talks about all the girls who are *silent and dead and still the life of the party*.

.   .   .

When I speak to Charlie in 2020, she finally feels as though she has left the incident with the vicar behind her. She has moved away from her old town and the old school she worked at and has started a new life in a new place. She no longer uses the BDSM website where she met her rapist, although she checks it sometimes, and she has noted that despite her making several complaints to the site, his profile is still active.

Charlie has found a new community that suits her desires and her sexual personality. Her new town has a large and very active swinging scene, with popular sex clubs that are approachable and friendly.

In the swinging community, people turn up to a sex club, either in couples or alone, and the club has comfortable rooms that you can go off into with whoever you meet and fancy on the night. Charlie likes this because if people are in relationships, they are always, always honest about it. They either bring their partners along, or say in the first few minutes of conversation that they are in a committed but swinging relationship. She feels safe in the knowledge that she will never again have to unknowingly have sex with someone else's husband, someone's father, someone's priest.

Her first visit to the swingers' club was a few months before we speak for the first time on Zoom. The club is stylishly decorated and very welcoming, she tells me. There's a main room where everyone can mingle, with a bar and a dance floor and comfortable places to sit, and then loads of breakout rooms where you can go to have sex with whoever you meet and like. She's been going there regularly, and she has found a wonderful community there. She's also one of the only single women who swing regularly – usually it's couples or single men – so the group admires her for living the exact sexual life she wants. That has helped her be proud of it, too.

.   .   .

For weeks, all I can think about are the words *burial* and *resurfacing*.

3

Six months to three years after:

- Inability to work
- Isolation
- Memory triggers
- Suicidal thoughts
- Substance abuse

CHAPTER ELEVEN

Audre Lorde said in the 2004 collection *Conversations with Audre Lorde*: 'Pain is important: how we evade it, how we succumb to it, how we deal with it, how we transcend it.'

Medical professionals and scientists have recently made a series of breakthroughs in the study of what is now known as chronic pain. Doctors define chronic pain as pain that has afflicted the sufferer for more than three months.

My own abdominal pain began in November 2009. That means for about eleven years, it has technically been chronic – rather than acute – pain.

Acute pain is the feeling that our culture usually associates with suffering. Acute pain is temporary. It is a broken ankle, a sports injury, a sore throat. It is a distress signal sent from a part of the body that is damaged up through the nerves along the spine and into the brain. When the physical problem is healed, the pain subsides. This is how we still, far too often, define and describe pain. For many people who live in pain, this narrative is achingly inaccurate.

When there is physical damage to a tissue or organ and the nerves receive these pain signals, the purpose is for us to act on them. Rest. Ice the injured ankle. Seek medical care.

But when those pain signals are sent and we do nothing, the nervous system becomes confused. It sends double the number of pain messages, then triple. Before long it is sending ten times as many pain signals to the brain, for the very simple reason that the regular amount is not having the desired effect; it is not keeping us safe. When we are ignored, we speak louder.

This is why many chronic conditions can have peaks and troughs in terms of the amount of pain the sufferer experiences. The body will cycle through routines of sending an inappropriate amount of pain messages to the brain just to get the brain to take notice. The body knows something is wrong, but the brain has learned that women are expected to cope with pain. As always, I have now learned, the body wins out in the end.

So if we are experiencing acute pain but do not allow it to heal, the nervous system will become overactive and send too many pain messages. But if *that* doesn't work, the neuroplastic brain actually creates a new neural pathway that is a constant pain feedback loop – it will mimic being in pain almost all of the time as a precautionary measure, because it cannot trust its normal alarm system to get us to act. So the pain becomes chronic – it exists in the brain as a constant warning sign, even when the actual tissue damage is healed.

Once pain is chronic – and this is the part that doctors are only just beginning to understand – it is not a symptom. It is its own disease. It is a neurological malfunction in its own right. It is not caused by a separate injury but is an injury to the brain itself. This makes it almost impossible to tackle.

So here's the kicker: ignoring the pain of women, trans and non-binary people does not only stop us from healing, it actually makes it more likely the pain will become permanent. Does that make you angry? It makes me angry.

Women are 25% less likely to be given opioids when they present to an emergency department with acute pain, as cited in 'Gender Disparity in Analgesic Treatment of Emergency Department Patients with Acute Abdominal Pain', a study published in the peer-reviewed journal *Academic Emergency Medicine*. When they are given pain-killers, they are given a lower dose than men reporting the same degree of pain.

Women in pain wait an average of sixteen minutes longer than men to be seen by a doctor, according to the *New York Times* piece 'When Doctors Downplay Women's Health Concerns'. When women go to a doctor with a painful condition, the pain is much more likely to be dismissed as psychosomatic or just a part of ordinary life.

This is why it takes an average of seven to ten years for a woman with endometriosis to be diagnosed and treated.

Elaine Scarry wrote in her book *The Body in Pain*: 'To be in pain is to have certainty. To hear that another person has pain is to have doubt.'

No one knows the feeling of being doubted better than a woman does.

The actual function of acute pain is not to torment us but to alert us to danger, Norman Doidge writes in his 2018 book *The Brain's Way of Healing*. With chronic pain, however, the alarm system has stopped working because the person responding to it has continued to override its messages, to insist that they do not deserve the attention it is demanding, to question the legitimacy of their own bodies. Is it any surprise, then, that so many patients of chronic pain are women?

As this pandemic rages while I write, I am thinking a lot about the language we use to talk about illness and pain. It is always a language of combat, of war. It is militaristic and individualistic and heavy with moral weight: those who survive pain and illness are 'fighters', endowed with some mystic property that entitles them to ongoing life. This language is not only masculine in its own right – in its violence – but also in the sense that it only imagines a definition of pain and illness that is *acute* and inherently *temporary*. The 'battle' is won, or it is lost. Either way, it ends. At some point, the fight is over.

Not so for so many women, too many. Not only are women much more likely to develop chronic pain conditions resulting from acute pain, but many of the hitherto untreatable chronic illnesses we contend with either primarily or exclusively affect women. For women, pain is not valiant and fleeting.

It strikes me that my illness was the end of a battle for me, not the beginning. I suffer deeply from my physical disability every day, of course. I'm not saying I don't struggle with it. I do. But not in the way that the word 'battle' evokes. That all came before. The battle was the lie: it was waking up every day and pretending I was something other than I was, pretending I hadn't been hurt by the world when I had. When I got sick, that was my body giving up on the lie. Illness was the most honest state in which I'd ever existed. In this way, it wasn't a battle at all. It was a relief.

As Frances, the protagonist in Sally Rooney's novel *Conversations with Friends*, says about her chronic illness:

> I realized my life would be full of mundane physical suffering, and that there was nothing special about it. Suffering wouldn't make me special, and pretending not to suffer wouldn't make me special. Talking about it, or even writing about it, would not transform the suffering into something useful.

Pain that does not end is not a high-energy battle or a fight to the death. It is the most boring, mundane experience on earth. It is simultaneously traumatic and dull. Something that should be extraordinary but, because of our lot, has become so very ordinary for women.

Everything about pain and illness that disadvantages women is even more debilitating for Black people, particularly Black women, and many racial minorities. Black women are significantly more likely to develop chronic illnesses than white women, according to a 2018 study by the University of California Berkeley, 'Racial Discrimination Linked to Higher Risk of Chronic Illness in African American Women'.

For too long we have made the mistake of believing that illness is caused by personal behaviour. After living through my own illness, and talking to so many people for this book, I'm convinced that this connection is imaginary. Illness is structural. The body breaks down

under the stress of structural oppression. As Sinéad Gleeson writes in
Constellations, 'the kingdom of the sick is not a democracy'.

.　　　.　　　.

I have just been given a GnRH injection by my gynaecological surgeon.
I have rampant endometriosis. It is very, very painful.

I am waiting for surgery to remove the disease from my body. It
will be my sixth endometriosis operation in eight years. I will have
to wait a month or two, but I am in debilitating pain, so my surgeon
has given me this injection to stop the disease in its tracks until the
surgery comes around.

The injection chemically induces menopause. It is a strong hormone treatment that freezes the menstrual system. Each injection
lasts one cycle. In theory, everything starts back up again after that.
Of course, there is always a risk that it won't.

For days now I have been having hot flushes during the night
and in the mornings. My mood is all over the place. I am irritable
and hungry. I am ashamed to tell anyone about my injection because
I don't want to admit that I might have sacrificed the one thing my
body is supposed to give the world.

The first time I meet Karolina, I realize that she is the first female
gynaecologist I have seen in the ten years I have been receiving
treatment for my endometriosis.

She looks over the surgery reports from my five previous lapa-
roscopies. I was diagnosed with endometriosis in 2010 after several
admissions to hospital through A & E with severe abdominal pain,
vomiting and bleeding. The disease is an inflammatory condition
involving tissue that is similar to the tissue that grows inside the uterus
growing in other parts of the body. The tissue grows and spreads on
the outside of various organs to which it does not belong – the kidneys, liver, bowels, and sometimes even the lungs and throat – and
causes a great deal of pain and internal bleeding. The disease causes
inflammation, and the cells form little tumours that bleed and burst

and weep. The foreign tissue, if left untreated, can build up and cause dysfunction in any of these abdominal organs, and can also cause infertility.

Karolina says I will have to have surgery. I think of the lines in Leslie Jamison's eponymously titled essay about struggling with illness, which appears in her collection *The Empathy Exams*. She writes:

> Getting your heart fixed will be another burglary, nothing taken except everything that gets burned away. Maybe every time you get into a paper gown you summon the ghosts of all the other times you got into a paper gown; maybe every time you slip into that anesthetized dark it's the same dark you slipped into last time. Maybe it's been waiting for you the whole time.

When Karolina looks up from her notes, she does something that no one – not a single one of my male specialists – has done in ten years. She explains to me exactly where the disease is in my body. She even draws me a diagram.

Because endometriosis remains under-researched and chronically misunderstood, there is no viable long-term treatment for the condition. Doctors do not know exactly what causes it or why, and are still undecided about whether it is an autoimmune condition, an inflammatory condition or a gynaecological one. Until the medical profession conducts more research and better understands the condition, the only intervention that provides long-term relief is invasive surgery to physically remove the damaged tissue from the body. I have had five such operations, and I am about to have my sixth.

There are two methods of surgery – excision and ablation. Excision cuts the diseased tissue out from the root, whereas ablation burns it away from the top. Excision is a much more difficult procedure, but a more effective one. Until my appointment with Karolina, I have no idea that the two types existed.

You have always had excision surgery, she says, looking over my surgical reports from 2009, 2010, 2012, 2013, 2015 and 2017. You've had the best surgery every time, and your disease has still grown back within two years. You are running out of options, she says, still kindly, still in her authoritative but reassuring tone.

I didn't know what she means, and I tell her so.

Well, she says, I don't know if you intend to have children, but my job is to keep your options open. And if you have many more operations, one of them will have to be a hysterectomy.

This is news to me too.

Each surgical procedure leaves scar tissues and masses of bloody, torn bits of leftover disease. Eventually, the scarring can become its own kind of dysfunction, an independent wound. Karolina says that you cannot keep performing surgery over and over because the scar tissue starts to damage the reproductive organs. At a certain point – and there's no telling when – the uterus has to be removed altogether. At this point – this was obvious, but in those moments in Karolina's office my mind is turning over itself very slowly – the window in which I could have children naturally will close. I would enter the operating theatre one day for my normal, two-yearly surgery and wake up barren.

Nothing taken except everything that gets burned away.

I cannot turn my mind to the real question at hand – whether or not I want to have children – to which I have no answers, only more questions. What strikes me instead is that Karolina is the first treating doctor I have ever spoken to who has not presumed that the role of the doctor is to keep intact my ability to reproduce naturally. My job is to keep your options open, she says. The most important thing is that when you make this decision, you have all the options to choose from. She wants me to be in control of my life.

Before meeting Karolina, several male gynaecologists had warned me about the impact of endometriosis on my ability to conceive, but they had done so in very different terms. Once, a doctor sat me down and said: Bring your partner in for the next appointment; we need to talk about how soon you can have a baby.

Sorry, what? I said. I was twenty-one and my partner was twenty-three. I did not want children – I still don't – but no one had asked me about this. Instead, my doctor said: Soon you will need to have a hysterectomy to treat your endometriosis, and if you want to have three kids, you'll need to have the first one next year.

I had never told my doctor I wanted three kids – I didn't – and I certainly hadn't told him I would be willing to have my first at twenty-two. I barely knew what to say.

When I protested, the doctor said: Well, you only have two options; it's that or we freeze your eggs for later, and that is very expensive.

(Children are very expensive too, no?)

You only have two options. In his world, the only alternatives were those in which my body was used to reproduce. That function was considered more important than the notion of my body being healed.

When I lift my eyes from where they are fixed on my hands in my lap, Karolina is drawing something. It is a diagram of the pelvic organs – the uterus, the kidneys, the small and large intestine, the cervix, the vaginal walls. On the left side of the diagram, she starts shading in whole swathes of the person's insides.

This is where your endometriosis has been found, she says, filling up more and more space with her pen. The kind of disease we have found is called deep incision endometriosis – it's the most deep-rooted form of the disease there is. It is very hard to remove.

As she is saying this name, she writes its acronym absent-mindedly across the top of the page.

D.I.E., it reads.

It says die, I say, laughing despite myself.

Karolina says they will do the surgery, but they will make it an extensive one. They will make sure nothing is missed so that I don't need to have another one for a long time. And after I recover from the surgery, they are going to try every way possible to stem the growth of the disease so that I have time to decide what I want to do with my body.

She tells me that she will put me on the urgent list and that they will do the best they can. She tells me that there is an injection she can give me that will help me cope with the pain and bleeding and inflammation between now and the surgery.

GnRH injections, or Lupron injections, are a form of hormone treatment that chemically induce menopause for one twenty-eight-day cycle. The hormones bring the menstrual system to a standstill for one cycle only, and once the twenty-eight days are up the drug wears off and the menstrual system continues to work as normal.

What this means is that the body will not produce oestrogen or progesterone at all in those four weeks. These two hormones are what fuel the growth and spread of endometriosis tissue, so halting their production will help to slow down the progression of the disease. The lack of hormones also means that the existing disease tissue does not inflame in the same way as it normally would once per cycle, so the injections can help a great deal with pain as well.

Many patients find huge relief in the treatment. I am sceptical, because in all my years of chronic illness I have been disappointed too many times to stay hopeful. I am the queen of false starts.

Doctors recommend that patients only use these injections for a short period of time, because the process of halting the hormonal system long-term can be very damaging. There is also a small chance each time you have the injection that the system will not start up again as normal, and the decision you made for the sake of a month's pain relief will become irreversible.

When I consult the internet and come across this warning, it brings me back again to the question Karolina had respected me enough to ask: do I want to have children? The answer is still no. Does that make me a monster? As this thought crystallizes in my mind, I think of Jenny Offill's novel *Dept. of Speculation*, how the main character says that she wants to be an art monster instead of a mother: 'My plan was to never get married,' she writes. 'I was going to be an art monster instead. Women almost never become art monsters because art monsters only concern themselves with art, never mundane things.'

Do I want to be an art monster? In any case, the treatment is short-term only. Karolina prescribes me three doses of the monthly injection and says that she hopes this will carry me through to the surgery, after which my pain will be much better managed due to the excision of the disease. I agree.

I cannot stop thinking about options. Jenny Offill writes: 'When God is a father, he is said to be elsewhere. When God is a mother, she is said to be everywhere. It's different, of course, for the art monsters. They are always elsewhere.'

I am surrounded by friends who are looking for ways to have a baby. People who have ended relationships because their partners didn't want them. I don't know why, but I've never felt so disconnected from the feelings of others. I cannot understand wanting to have children, no matter how much I try to stretch my imagination, no matter how much I try to occupy another's mind.

Two weeks later I am waiting in the gynaecology clinic at the Whittington Hospital. Normally, it takes months to get an appointment in this clinic, but Karolina has agreed to see me in between patients to administer my first GnRH injection. She walks out in between patients and ushers me in, chatting to me and asking about my pain management as she injects the long needle into my stomach and then deftly presses a cotton bud on the wound.

.   .

Sam was in her early twenties when she met Tim. She loved him, but she also knew, after not very long, that he wasn't good for her. That he was obsessed with being in control. He started telling her she was dirty and weak, a bad, rotten thing. She felt trapped by him, she didn't know how to leave, but she knew she was wilting in his presence.

Even when she did leave, Tim's voice stayed in her head. *You're nothing*, he would whisper to her in bed. Years later, when Tim's voice had faded, Sam realized her own voice was saying those things to herself, had picked up the slack.

Sam had two abortions while she was with Tim. When she recalls them now, she says she remembers them as though she was floating outside her body, looking in.

I suppose it was a way of minimizing pain, she tells me.

Sam had decided to go off the pill for a period of time and experiment with allowing her natural hormonal cycles to work unimpeded for a while. As so many of us have done since the option became available, she began tracking her cycle to identify when she was ovulating and when it was and was not possible to get pregnant.

There are only a few days in each month that it is actually viable to conceive a child, and natural cycles apps help you track those days and use condoms or stay away from sex during fertile periods. Sam explained this carefully to Tim, and he agreed to the plan. But then it was Sam's birthday, and he wanted to have sex even though she was fertile, and she agreed as long as he was extremely careful about pulling out, and then instead of pulling out he held her down and came inside her, and the next thing she knew she was pregnant.

I was upset, she tells me now, but didn't really know what to do about it, and it seemed petty to be angry with him, like he didn't understand what he had done.

Not long after, Sam had a surgical abortion. Surgical abortions are the kind most people would imagine – a hospital gown, a general anaesthetic. The alternative is a medical abortion, which involves taking a drug to induce the abortion at home.

Sam was already crying when she put on the hospital gown. We never talk about why, but I think I know. I cried when I put on my hospital gown for my abortion, too. If you'd asked me, in that moment, why I was crying, I might not have been able to answer you. I just was.

It just felt like that's what my body needed to do. Like it needed tears to process something my mind would not until years later, perhaps still hasn't, even now.

The doctors told Sam later that she cried the whole time; even when she was unconscious, the tears were running down even then, something that was happening in her body regardless of its interaction with her mind.

Afterwards I become extremely anaemic and kept on fainting, she tells me now. I also became really squeamish about blood, it was like every bit of blood I saw somehow felt like my blood, she says. I threw up once while watching Call the Midwife. I mentioned this to a friend at the time and they told me I needed to go to therapy, if I constantly felt like I was bleeding when I wasn't. I didn't go then, she said, but it did make me think about it.

When Sam got pregnant a second time, later in their relationship, two things had become clear to her. One was that Tim was abusive and narcissistic. The other was that she wanted a child.

I wanted to keep the baby this time, she said. I knew I wanted to. But by then I had finally realized how untrustworthy Tim was and I was terrified that the baby would be a psychopath, or would condemn us both to keeping Tim in our lives for ever.

So in the end, Sam knew she needed to save herself from her relationship more than she needed a baby. The two were mutually exclusive, and she had to choose the former.

With the memory of the surgery still alive in her body, the memory of breaking down during Call the Midwife as she tried to recover, the memory of everyone's bleeding feeling like her own bleeding, she decided to have a medical abortion the second time.

The chemical abortion is a weird experience, she tells me now, because you take one pill that stops your body from continuing to grow the baby, ultimately stopping life, and then you have to wait forty-eight hours before taking the flusher pill that expels it. It felt like I was carrying around my dead child for two days.

(I shudder at this thought. When I had my abortion, I found out too early that I was pregnant, at only three or four weeks, because I used to obsessively take pregnancy tests because I was so anxious, and then one of them just turned up positive one day. You cannot get an abortion before about six weeks, so I had almost three weeks of walking around knowing I was pregnant, knowing there was something growing inside me every single day, something I wanted dead. It was terrifying.)

When I took the flusher pill, Sam says, I was alone at our flat, and I was scared. I didn't know how much it was going to hurt, or how to tell if something had gone wrong.

Then she says: When it did finally start to happen, I nearly passed out from the pain. I know you understand that from the amounts of pain you have had to endure in your life, she says, and I nod.

It felt like someone was scraping my insides with a fork and setting fire to my spine, she adds.

I nod again.

My legs shook and I couldn't stand, Sam tells me, so I sat on the toilet with my face against the cold metal towel rail, now and again throwing up into the bath. It was such a mess, I wouldn't wish it on anyone. The only thing I could do was repeatedly say 'I can do this. I can do this. I can do this.'

I know the exact feeling she is describing. Curled up on the floor, inside a body screaming in pain and revulsion, completely alone.

After that night, Sam found it hard to deal with things like her period, or even smear tests. Everything became a reminder.

I used to use a Mooncup that I loved, and loved to be more ethical, she said. But I feel so uncomfortable with the idea of putting anything inside myself that I now just use pads, or tissue if there's nothing else.

The mantra Sam repeated to herself on the bathroom floor – *I can do this, I can do this* – was absolutely true. She could do it, and she did. But there was a cost. There always is for women and non-binary people. I think about all the times I have lain on a bathroom floor and whispered those words, hearing them fall on the same tired tiles night after night, and I realize now that every single time has cost me dearly, even though I have survived. It should not have to be this way.

Tim had said he wanted a baby, but he still didn't take the news of her pregnancy well. He became convinced Sam had done it on purpose, as a way to control him and his behaviour. So he stopped speaking to her altogether.

It was all very unhealthy, she says to me. But it showed me that I had to leave him, more than anything else ever had.

Then she says: So for that, I am grateful.

And then: It's kind of like creating new life in a different way.

And I smile.

Sam is a dancer now. Dance and movement have not always been an easy thing, she tells me. I was really, really shy as a kid and spent most of my time with all the animals I'd managed to get my dad to let me keep. The idea of people looking at me and at my body was the scariest thing. It still is sometimes. But I have always loved dancing, and in my teens I realized that it was one of the few things that made me actually present.

I felt the same way about my gymnastics, I think as I hear this. It was the only time when my mind was truly still.

Most of my memories as a kid I remembered by seeing myself do the thing, Sam says next. I didn't remember the actual sensations of doing.

Then she says: It felt like I was always just outside of my body, looking past my right ear or something. When I danced or was intensely physical, I realized that I was able to remember doing those things more fully, without watching myself do them. I still remember my younger memories like this, but once I started to train my body and pay attention to it, the memories start to mix it up. Now I can tell that I'm drifting into disassociation and becoming too internal when my recent memory starts to do this again.

It's only recently that Sam has been formally diagnosed with post-traumatic stress disorder and has started processing the abuse she suffered as a child.

Dancing helps, she says. I feel like dance has helped me claim my body. It actually makes me want to cry with gratitude thinking about it.

.   .   .

A week after my first GnRH injection, I start to feel better. I mean really feel better. The abdominal pain that has been mounting and haunting me for months has changed. Become duller. Something has finally managed to take the edge off.

As an experiment, I start going to a very relaxed yoga class every day that week on my lunch break at work. I make it there every day. Even though some days I am still weakened by pain and have to sit in child's pose for whole minutes while the others move, at least I am there. This is the first time I have managed daily exercise since I was seventeen.

The feeling is intoxicating. For weeks, all I think about is exercise. About how much energy I have when the pain is not as severe, about all the things I can do with my body now that it doesn't hurt so much. I start running on a cross-trainer at the gym every morning before I start work.

I know that I am lucky. I speak to several women during this time in my life who have had terrible experiences with GnRH injections. Women who have felt no relief from pain but who have borne the full weight of the worst symptoms of menopause. Night sweats, chills, hot flushes, severe mood fluctuations. Like anything with this misunderstood disease, it's a lottery. This time, I have won.

Karolina gives me two more injections, on a Monday four weeks apart, in between patients. A few weeks after the third injection, we do the surgery. It is 4 February 2020. Just weeks before London hospitals and ICUs and morgues will fill up with Covid-19 patients. Again, I am lucky. On this occasion, my body has been spared.

.   .   .

A few weeks later, I meet Olivia. We laugh a lot as we talk over Zoom, mostly because that's what you have to do when you have a shared tragedy. It feels like an impulse; it just happens. Relief, maybe. Or a need to make the other person more comfortable in the presence of our trauma. Probably both.

Olivia was twelve years old when she moved from Lagos to London. On the cusp of being a teenager, she moved from a Nigerian school where everyone looked like her to a British school where no one did.

Growing up in Nigeria, Olivia was used to having female friends that she could talk to about braiding her hair, about the kind of clothes they liked to wear, about the colourism they experienced from teachers and passers-by and crushes. But when her parents enrolled her in a majority-white boarding school in London, she lost contact with all of these lines of communication. When you lose this connection with others at such a tender age, it is very difficult to not lose connection with yourself at the same time.

For years now, Olivia has suffered from a sharp pain in her abdomen for one week out of every month. It is debilitating at times, and it comes back every few weeks like clockwork. This is not her usual period pain, although she gets that too.

She tells me she isn't someone who ever goes to the doctor. It's never been in her nature, really. Growing up in Nigeria, it wasn't common to see a physician for anything other than the most serious and life-threatening ailments, she says. So by the time she is a young adult in the UK, it does not occur to her at first to take her pain to a doctor.

But eventually, as the pain gets worse, she has to. By fourteen, she had started asking her GP about the debilitating abdominal pain she was experiencing, but no one would help her. Again and again, doctors assumed she had a sexually transmitted infection. When she told them about her lack of sexual activity, they just didn't believe her.

She learned, again and again, that the young Black body is so hyper-sexualized that she simply couldn't get a doctor to take seriously the possibility that her illness wasn't a consequence of her personal choices – even though she kept telling them otherwise. She describes this beautifully to me as the 'hyper-sexualization of Black girls in the

UK's medical system and the erasure of youth'. It's not just a lack of belief, she tells me, but an active urge to redirect blame.

She says that for her, all of these coalesced into something heartbreaking. A migrant from Nigeria who had been taught not to approach doctors, she was faced with another medical system that forced her to sit in rooms with white doctors who were uncomfortable discussing female bodies and who overtly blamed her for the fact that hers was failing.

Exhausted, she resolved to pay closer attention to what was happening inside her and try and work it out for herself.

Olivia measured her cycle and worked out that the pain was appearing each month at the exact time of her ovulation. Googling 'ovulation pain' and doing further research allowed her to understand the mechanisms in her body that were causing her discomfort. Her research also pointed her towards the best ways to manage the pain each month and stop it from interfering with her day-to-day life. Olivia tells me that she has gradually found a way to cope with the suffering on her own terms.

.　　.　　.

The truth is that, even if Olivia had been inclined to approach Britain's health system for help with her pain, it is unlikely she would have been believed.

Because of some oft-repeated racist fantasies dating back to the eighteenth century, too many doctors still believe that Black patients experience lower levels of pain than white people from an equivalent injury.

In the 1787 manual A *Treatise on Tropical Diseases; and on the Climate of the West-Indies*, a British doctor, Benjamin Moseley, claimed that Black people could withstand surgical operations much more than white people. This entrenched racism in medicine also led to the so-called 'father of gynaecology' testing out all of his methods on female slaves – without using anaesthetic or pain relief.

Every day, doctors invoke racial bias to discriminate against Black patients, particularly Black women, to systematically under-treat Black pain. A peer-reviewed study published in the *Proceedings of the National Academy of Sciences of the United States of America* in 2016, 'Racial Bias in Pain Assessment and Treatment Recommendations, and False Beliefs about Biological Differences between Blacks and Whites', found that Black patients are less likely to be given pain medications than white patients and, if given pain medications, they receive lower quantities.

Another peer-reviewed study, 'Ethnicity and Analgesic Practice', published in the year 2000 in the *Annals of Emergency Medicine*, found that Black patients were significantly less likely than white patients to receive analgesics for extremity fractures in the emergency room (57% compared with 74%), despite reporting similar levels of pain.

A 2013 study in the *American Medical Association Journal of Ethics*, 'Pain and Ethnicity', also found that Black and Hispanic people received inadequate pain management compared with white patients.

A 2016 study in the *Proceedings of the National Academy of Sciences*, 'Racial Bias in Pain Assessment and Treatment Recommendations, and False Beliefs about Biological Differences between Blacks and Whites', showed that half of the white medical students surveyed endorsed at least one myth about physiological differences between Black people and white people. One of these myths was that Black people's nerve endings are less sensitive than their white counterparts'.

The centuries-old belief in racial differences in physiology has continued to mask the brutal effects of discrimination and structural inequities, instead placing blame on individuals and their communities for statistically poor health outcomes. Rather than conceptualizing race as a risk factor that predicts disease or disability because of a fixed susceptibility conceived on shaky grounds centuries ago, we would do better to understand race as a proxy for bias, disadvantage and ill treatment.

Black patients are more likely to have other symptoms dismissed too, on top of pain. Studies have shown that the neurological and physical symptoms of lupus, a debilitating autoimmune disease, are systematically overlooked in Black patients, who have to languish without treatment or diagnosis for much longer than their white counterparts. This still happens despite the fact that we now know that Black women are at a significantly greater risk of developing lupus than are white women, and they are more likely to have severe complications if they do develop the disease.

. . .

A few weeks later, I meet Angela over Zoom. She is energetic and clever, and I immediately know we will get along.

In her first year of university, in London, Angela was violently mugged on the street while walking home. Her assailants stole her wallet and phone before punching her in the face and breaking her jaw.

The attack didn't register very strongly with her, she tells me. She convinced herself that she was fine. She didn't want to talk about it.

But she was offered counselling and victim support by the police to coach her through the process of reporting the assault. It was this insistence on the legitimacy of her harm that allowed Angela to open herself up to treatment for post-traumatic stress disorder, which then allowed her to receive care for the mental health conditions she had suffered as a teenager and continued to live with as a young adult. So much depends on who we appoint as moral gatekeepers.

Angela's mental health deteriorated after the assault, and she found herself jumpy and afraid. She struggled to get through the rest of her year at university, and in the midst of this started a new relationship with a man she had met online.

The relationship lasted a year or so, and the two became very attached to one another. But there were toxic elements, too. Angela knew that, but she wanted it to work.

That's why, she tells me, it was so hard for either of them to let go when they finally broke up. The relationships you fight the hardest for are the most devastating to lose – especially if you've been fighting for them alone. I know what it's like to hold on desperately to a toxic relationship with a man who has all the power.

They kept seeing each other after the break-up, kept sleeping together. It was consensual, but Angela also knew it was unhealthy. She tried to create a boundary and stick to it. She told him she didn't want to sleep with him any more.

The next time they met up, he pretended he was okay with this. They were going to have a final conversation about them, about what had happened. But he wasn't okay with it, and he took what he wanted from her.

This rape brought back symptoms of Angela's anxiety and PTSD from the attack. Everything is cumulative.

Angela had always known she was attracted to women, but she had pushed herself to date men. After the rape and the break-up, she decided to start casually dating women, to see how it felt to explore that part of her sexual desire. She spent several months going on dates and having great sex with women, never anything serious, and nothing ever stuck, but she knew immediately that this was the truest part of her sexuality. It felt like coming home.

When Angela felt ready to be in a relationship again, she knew she wanted it to be with a woman. She kept dating, but with an eye towards something more. That's how she met Aoife, on a dating app. The two have now been together for three years.

It was Aoife who sat on the bathroom floor with Angela when she was struck down one day with unbearable abdominal pain.

It felt like I was dying, she tells me, wincing at the thought.

I know, I say. And I really do know.

She collapsed from the pain and allowed Aoife to call an ambulance. In the hospital, doctors found that she had a severely contorted ovary that was pressing on the nerves in her abdomen like a knife, twisted and stabbing and malicious.

The doctors found that Angela's ovary was under attack by endometriosis. They removed the diseased tissue but, as with any endometriosis patient, they knew it would most likely come back.

Angela and Aoife have talked about starting a family. They want children.

But on reflection, she says to me now, I don't think I would ever actually want to be pregnant. I don't think I could stand it. I've had enough of that part of my body acting up. I don't think I could spend nine months thinking about it by choice.

When I ask Angela how she feels about her body now, she says it's complicated. She has started listening to it much more, she says, started to tune in to what it's saying in a way she hasn't been able to for a long time.

Since her surgery, Angela has also been diagnosed with fibromyalgia – a long-term, chronic condition that causes pain all over the body. Angela has persistent abdominal and chest pain. The day I speak to her about this, she has just returned from yet another stint in accident and emergency.

Fibromyalgia can cause pain anywhere, but a lot of women told me it often comes in the back, neck and chest. Doctors have no idea what causes it, but it is a disorder of the central nervous system, a disease that causes pain signals to misfire. All doctors know is that it is often triggered by a traumatic or stressful event, such as surgery or an attack, and that it affects seven times as many women than men. Sound familiar?

A doctor has recently told Angela that her pain and her endometriosis could be a symptom of her post-traumatic stress disorder.

.   .   .

Endometriosis UK says that one in ten British women and people with female reproductive organs suffers from endometriosis, but for each one of them it takes an average of 7.5 years for the disease to be diagnosed. These statistics are much, much worse for Black women in the UK, who are half as likely to be diagnosed with endometriosis as white women.

The fact that so many women and people with uteruses are left to suffer without diagnosis or treatment for so long is alarming to many endometriosis specialists. On top of this, when patients do get a successful diagnosis, the battle for relief continues almost unabated. Because the condition is under-researched and misunderstood, treatment options are extremely limited, and there is no known cure. And, as if that's not enough, we still don't know what causes it in the first place.

Back in 2010, when my doctors first suggested that my endometriosis could be linked to trauma, understanding that endometriosis may be one of the long-term effects of my sexual assault meant I was finally grasping one of the many possible causes of the elusive, debilitating disease that was ravaging my body.

Arvind Vashisht, a consultant obstetrician and gynaecologist at London's University College Hospital, told me that endometriosis, just like many lifelong conditions, including cancers, is caused by a multitude of factors that 'switch on' a particular autoimmune response and cause damaged tissue to grow and spread. But we don't know yet what causes that switch to turn on.

It could be connected to trauma and stress held in the body, as my own doctors have suggested and as is argued by doctors such as Michèle Albina Piérobon. In her 2014 study, Dr Piérobon found that 91% of patients with endometriosis had a history of one or more traumatic experiences. A recent study of 60,000 sufferers by Holly Harris, ScD, an ovarian cancer and endometriosis researcher at the Seattle-based Fred Hutchinson Cancer Research Center, showed a link between endometriosis and experiences of child abuse.

Another possible cause, Dr Vashisht told me, is something called retrograde menstruation – which is when menstrual blood travels the wrong way through the body and ends up in the pelvis.

But what doctors have discovered more recently thickens the plot even further. It's possible that many women have retrograde menstruation without developing endometriosis. The thing that causes the disease itself is the immune system's response to the foreign tissue – something going awry in the autoimmune system that causes the body to attack the cells as if they are external toxins, rather than part of the body. It's this line of thinking that is driving a growing body of evidence that endometriosis could be, more than anything else, a disease of the immune system.

I spoke to another endometriosis specialist about this – Dr Peter Barton-Smith, the founder of the Endometriosis Clinic at the Princess Grace Hospital in London – who said that it seems more likely than not that the key to understanding endometriosis is not the presence of the damaged tissue itself, but the immune system's overactive response to it. Dr Barton-Smith told me that he has noticed that a huge number of endometriosis sufferers also have an autoimmune disease, such as lupus, indicating that endometriosis may well be related to a problem with the immune system. This is certainly true for me – not long after I was diagnosed with endometriosis, I was also diagnosed with Crohn's disease, a condition that causes inflammation throughout the body as a result of the body attacking itself.

Even if we knew what causes the disease or how to effectively diagnose it, we cannot treat or cure it. As I mentioned earlier, the only treatment available to properly relieve the patient of endometriosis is to surgically remove all fibroids and tumours through one of two kinds of invasive surgery. Excision surgery involves cutting the damaged cells out from their root, while ablation surgery involves burning away the tumours and scar tissue superficially. Outside of surgical treatments, the only options for managing the disease are hormonal modifiers, often through the contraceptive pill, and generic pain management.

How is it possible that a disease that causes lifelong disability for so many women and people with female reproductive organs is so under-researched and poorly treated?

I asked Mathew Leonardi, a surgeon at McMaster University in Canada. He reiterated that he believes endometriosis should be treated as seriously as ovarian cancer – with the same amount of research funding, clinical trials, and a focus on patient well-being. There are many similarities between endometriosis and cancer, Dr Leonardi told me. These include the way the disease grows and spreads around the body and the extremely debilitating impacts it has on a patient's quality of life.

Dr Leonardi said endometriosis deserves the same respect that cancer receives, but instead most patients are left with inadequate treatment and disabling symptoms. When I asked him why, he said there are a number of reasons, but a big one is because the condition is not immediately life-threatening. While endometriosis is not a disease that typically kills a patient, it can certainly kill huge parts of a patient's life. The medical profession is not accounting for that.

He also told me that classifying endometriosis as seriously as if it were cancer would allow for much better surgical outcomes as well. The operations required to remove endometriosis – of which I've had seven – are incredibly complex and very similar to the process of removing cancerous cells, Dr Leonardi said. But, in order to qualify to remove ovarian cancers, doctors must have many years' additional training. This is not the case for endometriosis specialists, he told me. That means patients can opt for the surgical route and still not have all their damaged tissue removed or all their symptoms resolved as the surgery is extremely technically difficult and under-trained surgeons risk overlooking disease and failing to excise it.

Dr Peter Barton-Smith said he regularly sees patients who have been told after diagnostic procedures that they definitely do not have endometriosis. But when he reviews their surgical images, he can see nodules of disease that less specialized doctors have missed. This leads, he said, to an alarming number of false negative diagnoses.

I am extremely lucky to have had a relatively early endometriosis diagnosis due to my being white, middle-class, cisgender and with access to universal health. But I still feel ashamed of my pain after so many years of having it dismissed and delegitimized by doctors who, to be blunt, didn't believe what I was telling them. It is a shame I have internalized – there are days when even I don't believe that my extreme pain and disabling symptoms are real.

I have heard so many stories of women and people with female reproductive organs like me, with endometriosis and so many other conditions. Vaginismus. Fibromyalgia. Myalgic encephalomyelitis. Lupus. Rheumatoid arthritis. Fatigue. The only thing that connects them apart from the stories I hear about dismissal and disbelief is the fact that the vast majority of sufferers are women or people with female reproductive organs.

.　　　.　　　.

Sunita tells me that she found it difficult growing up Asian in Britain. Her family is from Malaysia and Pakistan, and she found herself feeling isolated from her English friends because of her family's hyper-conservative expectations of her. While her friends were experimenting with make-up and skimpy clothes, Sunita's mother would scream bloody murder at her every time she tried to leave the house with skin showing.

Both of her parents were incredibly strict in this regard. She wasn't allowed to wear what she wanted, and she was banned from wearing make-up. Next to her friends who had the freedom to do these things, Sunita started to feel as though there was something about her body that was shameful.

She had one aunt who was more relaxed about the way Sunita dressed, so she would spend as much time with her as possible. But her aunt's children were allowed to dress like teenagers and wear band t-shirts and hang out with their friends, and this sometimes made her feel even more alone.

This led her into a strange double life. She would put on conservative clothes every morning to go to school and when her parents would inspect them, they would approve. But she hid a plastic bag in her backpack containing a completely new outfit, one she would change into before she arrived at school. She would carefully apply make-up and brush her hair, arriving at school a totally different person from the one she left her house as. She would search all over for the most effective make-up wipes, and she would struggle to pull the layers of black mascara off her eyelashes on the bus home from school. Using this tactic, Sunita was able to craft a life for herself in which she felt close to her friends and didn't risk being punished by her family.

I did a lot of stuff in secret, she tells me. I modelled from when I was about sixteen onwards. Hiding where I was going gave me a false sense of validation. I always struggled to get jobs being Indian. I believe the model industry is still racist.

I really struggled living between two cultures, she adds. I wanted the blonde hair and green eyes, the boyfriend, the blonde body hair and short skirts. But now, she says, she wishes she could reach back in time and tell her younger self that one day she would be proud of her culture.

Sunita is now thirty-eight, but her mother still comments on the way she dresses. Since she married an Englishman, though, things have settled down. In their eyes, she tells me, her husband is now the one who is responsible for any shame she brings due to what she wears.

Before she came up with this strategy of changing and remaking herself every morning before school, the only way Sunita could validly express herself was through her hair. She loved her hair; it was beautiful and luscious and long. So years later, when she was diagnosed with ovarian cancer and lost all her hair to chemotherapy, she was devastated. Sunita's family was reticent about gossip that would spread in their community if word got out about her cancer diagnosis, so she wasn't able to talk about it or reach out for help.

I blew up like a balloon one night in February, she tells me. When I got to hospital, they had to drain eleven litres of fluid out of me. That same night, they took out my right ovary and my appendix.

Following that night, Sunita stayed in hospital for two months while the doctors tried to figure out what was wrong with her. After a long wait, the doctors said she had cancer. Sunita was thirty-three and, even though she wasn't thinking about children at the time, she did want to know what her options were.

You had a nine-centimetre cyst on your ovary that had burst, the doctor said. So everything has been contaminated. You barely have any eggs left to freeze.

Sunita went through fertility treatment immediately afterwards, but doctors said that they could not harvest her eggs; her remaining ovary had a large cyst on it as well. They only managed to freeze eight eggs.

·　　·　　·

I think so much about Sunita for weeks after our interview, about how her community made her feel ashamed of her illness. About how she didn't feel able to talk about being sick with the people who were closest to her. Illness and shame are still so bound together for so many of us.

One morning, years ago now, I was seized by acute abdominal pain and vomited for close to nine hours without reprieve. I desperately needed pain relief but I threw up everything I swallowed, including the anti-nausea medication. I could not hold down a single sip of water, so by the time I had entered my tenth hour of vomiting I was barely conscious from dehydration.

I asked my partner to take me to hospital, but he said it would be a waste of time. He said he had to go to his parents' house for Sunday night dinner and I begged him not to leave me alone in the apartment. He refused to cancel, and insisted that I come with him instead.

When we arrived at his parents' house, I was placed in a spare bedroom to wait until dinner was over. At one point, my mother called from London and demanded I be taken to hospital. Still, I was not. I thought about calling myself an ambulance, but I decided not to, because part of me – most of me – believed that the condition I was in was shameful, a failure.

Hours later, in the hospital, a nurse asked me why I had taken so long to get help. I said nothing. You could have died, she said. She placed a hand kindly on mine and asked me if I was safe. I blinked back tears, hoping she could not see the tectonic plates moving inside me.

It seems to me that to be a woman is to be expected to handle pain. And not only handle it, but handle it gracefully. Without making a fuss. Without drawing too much attention to herself.

It scared me so badly that the only comforting idea I could think of was: maybe it's not happening. I kept returning to this thought every time I felt myself starting to panic, as if going insane and hallucinating an alternate reality was less frightening than what was actually going on.

That's how Sally Rooney's protagonist, Frances, describes her relationship with her endometriosis in *Conversations with Friends*. I developed a very similar relationship to my own illness, and what I discovered after years of being ill is that disappearance bleeds. I was so determined to pretend my pain wasn't real that I drew people close to me who wanted to believe it too. In doing this, I handed them a potent weapon.

It was May 2013 and I was having major surgery for my endometriosis for the first time since I'd met this boyfriend. We were in that head-over-heels, dopey kind of love. We knew nothing about each other really, but we were obsessed with the shadows of one another.

I woke up from the surgery scared, and called him. He did not answer. I called again. He was supposed to pick me up from the hospital at 9 a.m., but he didn't show up. I called again.

Many hours later he appeared, smelling of damp, stale beer and day-old cigarettes. He looked as though he had not slept. He was bouncing around the hospital room like a jack-in-the-box. He was still high on ecstasy from the night before.

I swallowed my sadness at his lack of interest and we hobbled out of the hospital arm in arm. When it became clear that my many abdominal surgical wounds were too fresh for me to be walking, we found a wheelchair and he pushed me to his car.

When I asked him where he had been, he said he had arrived home late and slept through his alarm. Soon it came out that in fact he had not arrived home at all; he had slept at the house of the girl he had been sleeping with a few months earlier, before I had come along. I swallowed my sadness again.

A few hours later we were lying on my futon and he told me he was in love with me as he played with the gauze on my surgical sites.

What do you do with someone who lies to you and then tells you they love you on the same day?

I continued to be sick and he continued to ignore it. There was a time when I became so sick with Crohn's disease and the side effects of the heavy dose of prednisolone I was on that I could barely make it into work for months. I was forced to repudiate all my responsibilities: I had to hand over the last half of my teaching work for the semester, I fell behind in my own studies, I withdrew from family and friends and hid in my own despair. But even when I could not find the strength to move my legs long enough to leave the house all day, I would somehow muster it when he needed me. And he always needed me. No matter how much of my own life I gave up to my sickness, my role as his guardian was one I could not forfeit. I got sicker from the sleepless nights and the panic of it all.

Traumatized people are good in a crisis: a gift I never asked for but could not send back. Between his propensity to be unstable and my unshakable desire to prove just how much instability I could handle, we built an impossible life together. My life became a performance, a transaction, all because I was too ashamed to demand the help I needed from the people close to me.

Psychiatrists who specialize in the impact of chronic illness on relationships say that a happy union leads to better pain management.

They also say that as pain can sometimes be the body's way of asking for help when the mind cannot, patients in constant pain should be treated alongside their carers. Because it is likely that the pain is, in part, an expression of what they are not comfortable asking for. The body is a canvas; it reads *help me* when we know the words themselves won't work.

So therapists say illness management should be communal, it should involve both partners. But as a woman, I had always believed, without ever being told, that my ability to maintain a relationship depended on my keeping my suffering to myself. His burden, I always understood, was to be carried between us. Mine was to be carried alone. I never felt entitled to a communal approach to my illness. Between us, our commitment to this idea was so potent that it almost killed me.

'Intimate Relationships and Chronic Illness: A Literature Review for Counsellors and Couple Therapists', a 2017 research paper published in the *Psychotherapy and Counselling Journal of Australia*, found that intimate relationship distress has a bigger impact on women with chronic illnesses than men. I suspect I know why. Women are taught to see caring as communal, no matter how bad things get. Men are socialized to withdraw.

I keep coming back to that statistic: that 70% of all sufferers of chronic pain are women. That chronic pain is a disease born when acute pain is ignored. Could our illness be, in part, a product of our society's belief that we ought to care for others instead of ourselves? That unlike what we're told on aeroplanes, we must always secure our families' oxygen masks before our own?

Could it also be a product of our society's belief that male partners in heteronormative relationships should be the recipients of care and not the source of it?

There is a scene in *Conversations with Friends* that I have never forgotten. Frances is in A & E after being struck down by debilitating abdominal pain, caused by her endometriosis. Weakened by pain and dizzied by painkillers, she speaks to the man with whom she is in a relationship – in which the power dynamics are already imbalanced. Over the phone he asks how she is, but she will not tell him. He suspects she has been drinking. He asks again, and she lies.

Nick is on holiday in France and he chastises Frances for calling him at 2 a.m., afraid the other guests will see her name flash up on his screen. She writes:

> Are you drunk? he said. What are you doing calling me like this?
>
> I said I didn't know. My lungs were burning and my forehead felt wet.
>
> It's only 2 a.m. here, you know, he said. Everyone's still awake, they're in the other room. Are you trying to get me in trouble?
>
> I said again that I didn't know and he told me again that I sounded drunk. His voice contained both secrecy and anger in a special combination: the secrecy enriching the anger, the anger related to the secrecy.

As Nick becomes angrier, Frances starts to punish herself:

> I began to feel upset then, which was a better feeling than panic. Okay, I said. Goodbye. And I hung up the phone. He didn't call back, but he did send a text message consisting of a string of question marks. I'm in hospital, I typed. Then I held down the delete key until this message disappeared, character after evenly timed character.

I have spoken to so many readers who fume at this scene, who observe it with bafflement. Why wouldn't she tell him? I hear them say. But to me, that scene made perfect sense. There is nothing more terrifying than becoming more vulnerable in a relationship in which you already have very little power. There is nothing more terrifying than knowing that the person on the other end of the phone wouldn't come if you needed them, and that you would stay with them anyway.

Sometimes – most of the time – it's better not to ask. To paraphrase Lisa Taddeo in *Three Women*, if we don't ask for what we want, no one will ever see us not getting what we need.

.   .   .

Sunita had her first round of chemotherapy soon after she got her diagnosis. She tells me her body responded quite well, but it coincided with the London lockdowns. Sunita could not see her husband for a full week during the worst of it, while she was in hospital.

I felt so alone, she tells me. Since chemo, Sunita has been shielding from the coronavirus and has not been able to see her family or friends.

Sunita's doctors have been pushing her to get a hysterectomy so the cancer doesn't spread to her womb, but she has refused. Culturally, surrogacy is not an option for her, a fact which she accepts. So she needs to keep at least the possibility of becoming a mother.

She also had to go into medically induced menopause during the treatment.

I got early menopause, which is horrible, she tells me. You can't sleep, you have hot flushes and mood swings. I lost my periods, she says. I am now sterile. She has eight remaining eggs, frozen in a lab.

I felt hopeless, she says, as though my identity had been stripped from me. I felt that my feminine side, my chance to naturally conceive as a mother, had been stolen.

When I speak to Sunita the first time, hair loss is a possibility, but it hasn't happened yet. She tells me how proud she is of her long, thick hair, how much she doesn't want to sacrifice it to her illness. It feels like so much has been taken from me already, she says. I don't want them to take my hair. Long, thick hair is seen as such a source of pride in Asian cultures, she says. It's the only thing I feel I am allowed to be proud of, and I might lose it.

She doesn't know it during that interview, but Sunita will lose her hair. Within a few weeks, she will contact me again to say she is becoming increasingly distressed and chunks of hair have started coming out in her hands in the shower, clogging up the drain. It's happening, she says.

A few days later, we speak again.

I lost my hair a few days ago, she tells me. After I washed it, it was a matted mess. I was wailing and sobbing in the shower and felt like my world was collapsing.

She was due to have an appointment with a hairdresser who specializes in working with cancer patients, but it is now pointless.

Sunita messages me on Instagram the day she starts losing her hair. Of all the things she has been through, she says, this part is the hardest. She talks as though I won't understand this, but I do. I still grieve for silly items I've left behind in hospital wards, things I never needed but feel sad for purely because of their context. And none of those things were nearly as important to our identity as hair.

Sunita also caught Covid-19 while undergoing treatment for her ovarian cancer. What an unimaginable year.

When we speak, Sunita is still determined to become a mother. Despite the fact that cancer stole her ability to conceive naturally and Covid-19 stole her energy and drive, she's sure that she will get there.

I've always had a maternal instinct and longed to have a child to share experiences with, to shower with love, and to help them succeed in the world, she says. She is determined to use the eight eggs she had frozen before her many operations to eventually have a child.

When I speak to Sunita now, she tells me how much shame is still attached to illness in the Asian community in 2020. No one is allowed to talk about it. When she first got sick, her mother begged her not to tell anyone. To her mother, it felt like weakness.

I want the Asian community to realize that cancer isn't something you should hide or brush under the carpet, Sunita says.

.   .   .

After my last hospital incident, I realized that my partner's determination to dismiss my illness was putting me in harm's way. A mentor told me I had to leave. I knew she was right. I will give you my life in every conceivable way, I remember thinking, but I will not die for you.

I got on a bus home and clicked on the first last-minute hotel booking site that came up on Google. I booked a room and packed my bag.

The research I mentioned above on chronic physical illness and intimate relationships also shows that, over time, an unsupportive partner can degrade the patient's parasympathetic nervous system. That's the part of us that regulates emotion, and being in a near-constant deregulated state wears down the nervous system. It contributes to heart problems and immune problems in the chronically ill. Being with someone who cannot cope with sickness makes you sicker.

I cannot tell you how many times I told myself that if I just got better, or managed the pain better, he would love me enough to care for me. To *want* to care for me. That if I stopped needing his help, he would offer it. How many times I told myself that my inadequacy was the problem, and that I could fix it, fix myself, make myself loveable, if I just kept trying.

But here's the thing about chronic illness: it is permanent. It cannot be fixed by trying harder, or by being kinder, or wanting wellness more desperately. It cannot be erased by dedicating oneself wholly to another body in the place of one's own. I had to learn that lesson so many times.

As long as there is someone with the power of proximity telling us that a diagnosis is a personal failure, something for which we alone are responsible, something we have an individual duty to overcome, we will stay in this alternate universe forever. It makes me think of a line in a poem I once read, called 'Holy Thank You for Not', by Megan Falley: *There are so many ways to die. Most of them you can do while living.*

I used to think that I was incapable of intimacy because of my illness. Now I know that there was only one person in each of my relationships who failed at intimacy, and that person was not me.

Erasing illness is a powerful weapon and one that is the most devastating when used by those closest to us. In this way, it is singularly cruel. It is also the refuge of those who are desperate for control, those who fear uncertainty. It is this quality of the need to erase sickness, I have realized, that should make us the most afraid. It is them, not us, who lack courage. Anne Boyer writes in her memoir, *The Undying*:

> The ones who have abandoned you, who – now that you are sick – have ceased to speak to you or come around or just say outright that they can't handle it, say that your illness, as they say, is 'too difficult' for them, have a hand at creating your existence, at least partially as someone who will always, at least in part, stay well.
>
> To them you are static and permanent.
>
> The people who left won't watch you suffer or diminish, so you are, by their actions, kept forever as you were at the moment of diagnosis.

Now I know what failing at intimacy really looks like. It looks like keeping score. It looks like wielding power over someone who is vulnerable. It looks like disappointing the person you promised to care for. It looks like walking away when you are most needed.

When the female body hurts, we do not listen. When the female body bleeds, we do not listen. These ancient signs of trouble have come to apply differently to us. As Sinéad Gleeson writes in *Constellations*:

> The shedding of blood has historically been seen as a male act of heroism: from rite-of-passage fistfights, to contact sports and combat. Infrequent, random events seen as standalone milestones; stories to tell once the pain – and enough time – has passed. Female bleeding is more mundane, more frequent, more getonwithit, despite its existence being the reason that every single life begins.

Ever since the Enlightenment, Western society has taught us that value exists primarily in the rational mind; that is, the conscious mind, the one in which we can deploy logic and reason and solve problems through human cognition. This kind of thinking, of course, has given us all kinds of exciting developments. But the determination with which we cling to the idea that logical thought is the only kind of intelligence we should listen to has shown itself to be very dangerous. It has transformed from a dedication to rationality to a dedication to thoughts at the expense of feelings.

The realm of conscious thought encourages us to stop listening to our emotions, which are felt in the body and experienced by the mind long before they are transformed into rational thoughts. So by only listening to the final product – the thought, with its logic and reason and informed by all we know about the body – we lose some of the most important information available to us about ourselves: our raw emotions, our intuition. It is a significant loss that we have developed into a society that considers feelings last.

It's also not a coincidence that the kinds of intelligence we value are broadly masculine ones: they prioritize formulaic reasoning and the notion of individual rights over relational thinking, they tend to devalue emotional responses as weak or irrelevant. Because men led the Enlightenment and every society that followed it, they wrote themselves into all of the foundational aspects of our society. They built their own qualities into our universities, our science labs, our governments and our laws. I hope this is changing, and some days I think it is, but it still seeps into my life regularly. Emotion as weakness. Rationality as strength.

This means that we are conditioned to distrust or undervalue the kinds of intelligence that are more associated with femininity – emotional intelligence, the ability to understand others in relation to the self, intuitive intelligence and embodied knowledge. Most importantly: pain.

We are so far down this path that we have altogether stopped listening to our bodies and what they tell us about how we *feel*, rather than just what we *think*. We walk around as floating heads.

My repeated misdiagnoses when I first got sick after my rape were a product of this same kind of thinking: my symptoms did not fit a formula, and the primary symptom – pain – is treated as outside the realm of science and devalued because it is a feeling.

My pain held more information about my condition than anything else, but no one was paying attention. It was screaming at us and we were ignoring it, too busy poring over blood tests that might *prove* something. The proof was there all along, but we missed it.

All because no one was listening to my body. Even me. *Especially* me. If I had listened, would I have been heard? I'll never know.

.   .   .

Olivia had always had perfectly clear skin, ever since she was a girl, and all the way through puberty and her teenage years. It had always been something she had felt incredibly confident in. It was one of the things she never questioned about her body, she tells me.

I always knew I could go make-up free if I needed to, always had a sense that where my face was concerned, I had nothing to hide, she says.

But something changed in her mid-twenties. Around the time she developed pain in her stomach every month, Olivia noticed that her skin become littered with pimples and craters, out of nowhere. It was like a second puberty, she says.

Olivia's new skin caused her confidence to plummet. Along with her pain, it felt like something fundamental inside her body was starting to go wrong. She hated having to cover her face in make-up every day just to go to work, knowing that her newly bad skin would cause people to look at her differently.

But the way her skin looked wasn't the worst part. It hurt, it itched, she said. It caused her to scratch and scratch until she had dug craters out of the flesh, like something was trapped under there that needed to get out.

.   .   .

How to conclude a chapter about pain? Pain is a slew of paradoxes. It is boring and yet intense. It is passive and active. It is so nebulous that it defies both language and definition, but at the same time it is also very specific. It is acute and chronic. It is a symptom *and* a cause.

CHAPTER TWELVE

I told you earlier in this book that I have spent the last ten years in and out of hospital, suffering from pain, abdominal bleeding, vomiting and loss of consciousness that was eventually diagnosed as endometriosis and Crohn's disease. I also told you that there is a growing body of research that suggests that these long-term conditions, as well as multiple sclerosis, fibromyalgia, diabetes and some cancers, could be the consequence of damage caused to the body by long-term post-traumatic stress disorder.

What that means for me now is that I live with two invisible illnesses that are, on most days, debilitating. It means I'll never know whether, on any given day, I will be able to work or not. Whether I'll be able to eat or not. Whether I'll be able to sleep, exercise, socialize. As awareness rises around just how devastating these conditions can be, we have started to develop a new language to explain what it's like to have a condition that is physically disabling on some days but not others. We call them invisible disabilities, or dynamic disabilities, because on some days you can see them and some days you can't. A lot of people with my conditions have wheelchairs and canes that they use on bad days, and I'm thinking about getting myself some as well.

I'm telling you this because I have recently discovered an amazingly helpful community of disabled friends online, and I have been speaking to them about this idea of the 'cool girl'. About how even though that pressure to be effortless, to be *chill*, to be unflappable, affects all women, it is so much heavier for those of us with disabilities or severe health conditions, because we know that those illnesses make us seem so very vulnerable. There is nothing cool or chill about being rushed to an emergency room.

So when I interview Dale for this book, and she says to me that she tries to be brave and untouchable to compensate for her disability, I know what she means. I do it every day. Every romantic partnership I've embarked on in the last ten years has begun with an elaborate performance from me, a stage play of a girl who is ethereal and spontaneous and agreeable and rarely prickly. I try extra hard to be that girl because of how deeply I know she will never be real.

There's another layer to this lie as well, one I've only recently uncovered. Dale mentioned it to me too. It's that there is a fundamental part of the 'cool girl' myth that is about the pressure to not need anything from a romantic partner. The pressure to be self-sufficient. The pressure to never depend on anyone, to never become attached.

There are so many tropes that tell us again and again that we have to be the 'cool girl' in order to be loved. That we have to not text back, never cry, never feel alone, never need help.

I know that the needy girl in the romcoms never gets the life she wants, and that is terrifying for me because my illness means that I *really* need people. It is hard not to be needy when there are days your hands don't work and your legs can't hold your body upright.

This applies to the healthy as well as the sick. It is a toxic expectation placed upon women. Even before I got sick, I put all my effort into pretending I was more independent than I am.

.　　.　　.

When she was eight, Dale started learning to read lips. She found that it helped with making friends at school when her hearing aids were patchy or unreliable, and the new skill made her feel a bit like a superhero.

Dale started wearing bilateral hearing aids when she was seven years old. She was born with hearing difficulties, but they didn't require intervention for the first few years of her life. Hearing was difficult for her as a toddler, but it was manageable. The condition deteriorated as she got older, and soon the hearing aids were a necessity. With them in, she could hear some things. She could vaguely hear the ocean, but she still needed to read lips every day.

Her strongest memory of childhood is people telling her they were sorry she was deaf. She hated it. She would constantly tell people there was no need to be sorry. She didn't want to be different. She knew she was deaf, but she didn't want anyone to be sorry about it. She just wanted to be normal.

She adopted a ruthlessly sunny disposition to try and counter this effect, Dale tells me. She wanted all the grown-ups around her to know that she was *fine*. That she didn't need their help. That she was happy and healthy. This way she felt less visible.

I'm just so sorry that you can't hear the ocean, her mother said once on a family holiday to the seaside.

The comment broke Dale's heart, and she redoubled her commitment to the pretence that she was unbothered by her disability.

I was so determined for it to never make a difference that I wound up putting the rest of my body under more pressure to compensate for my disability, she tells me in 2020.

Dale's way of outrunning her disability, she tells me, was to try and be brilliant at absolutely everything she did, so that no one would notice her impairment.

Whenever adults noticed Dale coping well with her deafness, they would use the word 'brave'. So she started associating bravery with impenetrability; with infragility. That's all she wanted to be. A girl who was untouched by emotion or difficulty. A brave girl.

This became a way of life for her. Throughout high school, she dedicated herself to her studies as ferociously as she had dedicated herself to learning to read lips. She excelled at everything she did. This was the best way to hide in plain sight.

By the time Dale was a teenager, this attitude had bled into the way she thought about sex and relationships too. She could see all around her that the way to succeed at intimacy as a teenager meant being detached from her emotions. It meant being the cool girl. She studied this, too, and she perfected it.

In the name of brilliance, she says to me, I wanted to be the coolest, *chillest* deaf girl. To me – and here she pauses to say *unoriginally* – that meant being slim, acerbic, kissing boys, and drinking beers.

I nod furiously again. All the ways we are taught to separate ourselves from our bodies and from our emotions eventually coalesce, I think. A perfect storm.

Halfway through Dale's first year of university, she suffered her first real heartbreak. The first boy she fell in love with left her unceremoniously, and she had never felt so alone. Living in first-year halls surrounded by other freshers, she didn't know how to process the feeling, so she decided she would avoid processing it altogether.

The heartbreak and her determination to run from it left Dale with an eating disorder that stayed with her for four years. She developed crippling anxiety alongside her new punishing eating habits, which eventually turned into severe depression and suicidality in her early twenties. This then turned into a misdiagnosed physical illness that lasted for months and months.

Not cool or chill, she tells me. But at least men still complimented my legs.

After the break-up, Dale continued to seek normality by getting men to fancy her, to outrun the pain in her chest and the numbness in her ears.

I was so busy being defensive about not needing special dispensation or help, she says to me, that I couldn't see how exhausting and time-consuming it is to be constantly adjusting one's posture to see someone's lips; to spend social evenings trying to grasp and guess the topic of conversation, trying to keep up; to do this while also just being a regular, stressed, heartbroken undergraduate. It's really very basic, isn't it? she says, and I nod and laugh again, feeling more connected to her by the minute.

At the height of her self-loathing, Dale realized that drinking took the sharp edges off the way she felt about her body.

I thought alcohol would keep me slim, she says. But perhaps more importantly, the hazy drunk gaze was kinder to her than her sober one; it dulled the harshest thoughts.

I drink for the same reason, I think – it numbs the most vicious parts of me.

My drunk gaze made me feel hotter and more confident, Dale says. Plus, alcohol calories feel less real than calories in food.

Ha, I say to myself. I know that trick, too.

.   .   .

I was sitting in a Thai restaurant in North London one evening, waiting for my green curry to appear. I had just broken up with Alex, the boy I had met on a dance floor. I tuned in to a couple sitting near me who were clearly on a first date.

She was quick-witted and clever, making dry jokes about the news and picking up on threads from conversations they'd had earlier in the night. He seemed impressed. So was I. I noticed her mention a few things that told me she had a very interesting job, a TV journalist of some sort, though her date never asked her for more detail, so I was left hanging.

What I did get, though, was reams and reams of information about him: his life, his football team, his friends, his mother. She nodded along and politely interrupted with sharp follow-up questions, the kind that made him seem interesting just by the fact of her asking them. Questions designed to cast the glow of her mind onto his.

He was talking about start-ups and sales strategy and explaining how his boss was useless, which was irritating, he said, but mostly he felt sorry for her. That was big of him, I thought.

The waiter came over to tell me that my bill was ready, but I was hooked. I asked him if I could sit a little longer.

He was asking her what kind of men she usually dated. She started to answer, said something about kindness, but he interrupted her before too long to present a soliloquy about how he just needed someone who wasn't too emotional, wasn't too dependent, who wouldn't get jealous when he went to the gym. So many women he met on these dating apps were *just a bit needy, you know?* he said.

She started explaining that she was independent, that she was busy, that she didn't have much time for dating anyway so that wouldn't be a problem.

It was the first time she'd been asked a question in the forty-five minutes since I'd been there, and she had to use it to defend herself against an accusation that she hadn't had a chance to do anything to deserve.

The first time she was allowed to hold space on the date, she had to use it to address a need of his: his need to be reassured that she would never need him, his need to feel protected by her ability to not need his protection, his maddening and obsessive need to depend on her to tell him she would not depend on him.

I have witnessed so many versions of this conversation, and I have participated in many more. I wish I could get those hours back.

Briallen Hopper's title essay in her collection *Hard to Love* is about learning to pry herself away from love that drained her, from a man who emptied her. She offers the fable of the crane wife.

In the story, she writes, there is a crane who tricks a man into thinking she is a woman so she can marry him. She loves him, but she knows that he will not love her if she is a crane, so she spends every night plucking out all of her feathers with her beak. She hopes that he will not see what she really is: a bird who must be cared for, a bird capable of flight, a creature, with a creature's needs. Every morning, the crane-wife is exhausted, but she is a woman again. To keep becoming a woman is so much self-erasing work. She never sleeps. She plucks out all her feathers, one by one.

Hard to Love is about dependence, about this promise women make that they will not depend, about the emotional test designed for them to fail, about the hot shame women feel when they do. And they always do.

She describes all the effort she goes to just to seem detached and un-needing to someone who considers himself too good for dependence. For someone who considers himself unbothered by human needs.

She writes about her own boyfriend, for whom she performed this not-needing. She describes how he aspired to be like Ralph Waldo Emerson, who wrote about the self-reliant man, who wrote this three-word manifesto for the independent male hero: INSIST ON YOURSELF.

I have never read a phrase that better captures every romantic relationship I have been in. Men who, when faced with any decision, repeat this phrase like a prayer: *Insist on yourself. Insist on yourself. Insist on yourself.*

The self-made man: the man for whom we have to pretend we do not feel, do not need, is, as Hopper describes him, 'simultaneously entitled, dismissive, and hard to get'.

Emerson believed that emotional dependence is the birthplace of shame. There is shame in being an object of empathy, he thought. There is shame in capitulating to requests for help. A man ought to be able to withstand any degree of pain without the need to be soothed.

Reading this, I realized that Emerson's self-made male archetype had seeped into my own belief system. Ever since I could remember, I had been convinced that there was shame not only in watching another person capitulate to my requests for help, but that there was shame in making the request at all.

In my romantic life, I learned not to ask for help because I believed, without ever being told, that in all likelihood the men sitting opposite me would see this as weakness. Eventually, I started to see it as weakness too. I was wrong. Asking for help is a formidable display of strength.

Being taught that we must suppress our emotional needs is toxic, it bleeds. Before long we believe that we must not need help in any aspect of our lives, that we must fashion ourselves into hyper-competent, unshakable superwomen in order to be worthy of love.

Hopper writes: 'For years I lived with the knowledge that if I ceased to be a successful, self-motivated, ambitious, size-six Ivy

League blonde, I would lose love. And I knew I couldn't live without love.'

I admire this in her, because I didn't have that kind of conviction. After a while, I couldn't stand the shame I felt when I admitted that I had needs, and I couldn't argue with the voice in my head that said that love depended on invulnerability, so I started to believe I did not need love at all.

I don't need anything from anyone, I'd been saying, again and again, for months, because I was tired of not having my needs met and I wasn't brave enough to expose myself to the same chasm of compassion again and again. So I retreated from love, and I told anyone who would listen how brave that was. How I just didn't need help from anyone.

Emerson thinks every man is entitled to be an island. I used to think that, too. So, as Hopper writes, 'my desire to twine like a vine was constantly thwarted by a man who was always carefully disentangling himself.'

This imagery is poignant; the tearing away of vines that need to interlink in order to climb. There is nothing more rupturing than the feeling of watching someone pull away when you need them. The feeling of knowing they are retreating not in spite of this being the moment you need them to stay, but because of it.

I decided some time ago that I was someone who could withstand any degree of harm without the need to be soothed, because it was the only way to protect myself from the people who refused to soothe me. From the men who insisted, again and again, on themselves, and who thought that capitulating to someone's need for help was the same as giving a part of yourself away.

And so women learn to lie. Women learn to perform self-reliance in his image just so that he will not leave them as punishment for the fact of being human, the fact of having human needs, the fact of not being an emotional island. Hopper perfectly captures how absorbing this project can be: 'I depended on his demand that I not depend. I leaned on not leaning on him. The irony was he left me anyway.'

The paradox of dependence is that men tell women in big and small ways that they cannot bear the thought of themselves depending on their female partners, so women perform non-dependence because it is the only way they can hold on to that human need for connection. For women, this performance is a prerequisite for love. And because women are human, and because they have needs, they need love just like everybody else does.

I use the phrase 'non-dependence' here because I need to make desperately clear that we are not talking about independence, not really. 'Independence' is the wrong word for this evasive quality women are taught to chase. It is not independence at all because true independence is inward-looking and self-defining. What is being asked of women here is wholly dreamed up by others.

Performing non-dependence is not about women at all, but rather about reading him carefully enough to know exactly what kind of un-needy-ness he – ironically – needs.

Hopper writes: 'We are far too prone to punishing ourselves and others for needing something we cannot exist without.'

The truth is that the woman being described by the boring man in the Thai restaurant is not an independent woman, or a 'calm' woman, or a self-sufficient woman, although these are the words he will use to talk about her.

No. She is not a woman at all. She is a mirror. An inanimate thing that needs nothing from him but has an endless capacity to reflect back his favourite parts of himself. Someone whose questions reflect his existence in a way that makes him feel interesting and special and worthy of not being needed by such an impressive, clever girl.

Because here's the other thing about the 'cool girl'. Her performance of non-dependence not only makes him feel safe but it also makes him look good. He is the man who gets to pretend to be unthreatened by the powerful, self-sufficient woman while using the

266 · LUCIA OSBORNE-CROWLEY

same narrative to keep her in a stuffy, windowless box in the space
between genuine connection and true independence.

She must behave like a 'real woman' so he can see himself as someone who is partnered with such a woman, but she must never actually be one. She must perform a non-dependence that is, in theory, threatening so he can be the special man who is not threatened, but she must never actually threaten him.

While he demands that she need nothing, he is in truth manifesting the greatest dependence of all: using someone else's life to justify your own.

He pretends he doesn't want committed love, but he does. In fact, he wants a superlative kind of love: a romantic partner who is so committed she can tend to all his needs while tending to her own and also find time to perform the not-needing he needs in order to feel brave enough to be loved by her.

Just writing these sentences makes me feel exhausted. I have played this role for years of my life, and I have seen the women around me play it, too.

But I don't want to be loved by someone like that. If that's the prize, I am not interested.

The work of becoming a woman worthy of this particular kind of heteronormative romantic love is itself a paradox. You work for years building something, not outwards or upwards, but inwards: building yourself smaller and smaller, with erasure as the ultimate goal. All to become something you never really wanted to be.

And what's worse, you will always fail, because pretending to be unhuman, with no human needs, is unsustainable. And when you do, he'll be waiting to punish you for splintering his fantasy. The irony was, he left me anyway.

Emerson wants men to know that 'they are not leaning willows, but can and must detach themselves', Hopper writes.

The woman in the Thai restaurant was visibly anxious now, acutely aware that he had undermined her and made her feel small. As she walked to the toilet, he got this look on his face. Like he knew he was supposed to feel guilty, but he didn't really care.

Every morning, the crane-wife is exhausted, but she is a woman again. To keep becoming a woman is so much self-erasing work. She never sleeps. She plucks out all her feathers, one by one.

To keep becoming a woman is so much self-erasing work.

I will not be the 'cool girl', the dream girl, the crane-wife, because she is a lie. She is a straw-woman in a field full of hungry ravens, and I am done with her. She's not worth it, and neither is he.

.   .   .

It wasn't until later in her life that Dale realized she was attracted to both men and women, and she now has a long-term girlfriend who doesn't even think her legs are her best feature. She tells me she loves her body now, and that her ability to identify as disabled and queer has been a huge part of that process.

I don't wear it as a badge of honour, but I do tell people now and ask them for help, she tells me. I don't want people to be 'sorry' that I'm deaf: I want them to believe me, and to do some of the work with me. More broadly, I feel I own my body now too, and I listen to it and feed it, she says.

Another thing Dale tells me about learning to love her body, something I have heard from a number of the people I interviewed for this book, is about getting sober. When we speak, Dale hasn't had a drink for three months.

I decided to just 'stop for a bit' after a boring wine hangover from celebrating a friend's birthday on Zoom, she tells me. I handed my girlfriend a bowl of egg fried rice, tofu steak and soy cucumbers for breakfast, and asked her how she'd feel if we quit for a bit.

They had both tried getting sober before – once as a New Year's resolution, once for Lent.

Ultimately, however, I kept drinking every night, she says to me, and kept being just a tiny bit or a big bit hungover every morning, because it was a habit, and I hated the idea of admitting that I couldn't handle it.

Another 'cool girl' move, I think. An invisible prison.

The idea of getting sober felt shameful, she says, because it would mean admitting that it had been a low-key problem for years, and that she had prevented it from becoming a big problem only because of her ability to cope and to present a functioning facade.

Eventually I began to crave sobriety, she says, I truly longed for it, but I didn't know how to do it when drinking was so ingrained in my personality, my evenings, my rewards.

Then, on this random Thursday, she tells me, it somehow stuck.

I've learned that this is true about so many things related to recovery: you just have to keep circling back to the same thing, the same step forward, again and again, getting a little bit closer every time, trusting that one day it will work.

Dale adds: I describe that Thursday morning hangover as 'boring' very deliberately because I really was bored of hangovers. Bored of the dry eyes and dehydrated, aggravated skin and bloated belly and stomach cramps and, sometimes, the shaking and the blackouts and the low, low moods.

I nod. I know this feeling.

.   .   .

Almost every day since I had disclosed my rape, I had spent the evenings drinking until I passed out. I used to drink until I didn't know where I was, or who I was, or what had happened to me. I would wake up bleary-eyed and sick and shaking but at least I would have forgotten what it feels like to have someone wrench themselves inside you with a blade to your throat.

I had a drawer full of OxyContin from my years' worth of surgical procedures and hospital stays, so I started taking them when I felt so sad that I couldn't breathe. I took more and more and more of them as the days went on and the process of healing didn't get any easier.

There was a night when I drank two bottles of red wine and took four Ambien and woke up fourteen hours later covered in vomit. I had thrown up all over myself and I hadn't woken up while it was happening. I almost killed myself that night. Not intentionally, not really. But this is the thing I've learned about suicide. It's not always dramatic or even intentional. Sometimes it's a slow, stumbling thing. Sometimes it's just the clumsy build-up of habits you learned from months and months of desperately not wanting to live. Sometimes it just comes from wanting to die for so long that one night you forget to save yourself.

All these months of self-medicating were driven by the belief that if I just waited for more time to pass, if I just got myself to the next day, to the next appointment, eventually it would get better.

It didn't. Time does not heal all wounds. There are some things you cannot just live through. You have to feel them. Really, really feel them. Feel them until the feelings run out. As my best friend says: the only way out is through.

The only way out, I discovered, is in.

It was a bright Sydney winter's day when I realized this. The sun was coming up over my apartment. I had been awake all night even though I'd taken sleeping pills. I was wondering why I hadn't been able to fix myself yet.

And then I found a passage from Cheryl Strayed's article, 'Tiny Beautiful Things':

'Most things will be okay eventually, but not everything will be. Sometimes you fight really hard and you lose. Sometimes you hold on and realize there is no choice but to let go. Acceptance is a small, quiet room.'

I don't know why, but something shifted inside me when I read those words. Something stilled. Something breathed in and out and in again. I had never felt more connected to another human being than I did in that moment. Cheryl understood something about me that I had been trying desperately to run from: I couldn't undo what had been done to me. I could try to live with it, but I couldn't erase it. No amount of alcohol or drugs or dates or parties could do that. I would have to rebuild myself around it. Most things would be okay eventually, but not everything would be.

After that day I started doing this as a ritual: picking up a book when I felt desperate, just in case this same magic happened again. And it did.

I have had a copy of Leslie Jamison's first essay collection, *The Empathy Exams*, in my bedside drawer since I first read it in 2015. It's thumbed and marked up and dirty and it makes me feel good just to hold it. One day when I was thinking about hurting myself, I pulled it out and started reading from the last essay in the book, called 'The Grand Unified Theory of Female Pain': 'The pain is what you make of it. You have to find something in it that yields. I understood my guiding imperative as: keep bleeding, but find some love in the blood.'

I had that feeling again, like something had stopped spinning inside me. Like something desperate had suddenly let go. It was only for a moment, but it was enough. The destructive impulse in me had passed. Not because anything about my life had changed, but because Leslie was bearing witness to it. Because she could see me, and I her, and I understood in this moment that she had been where I was, and that she had held on. She had found something that yielded, and she had made something of it. And the thing she had made was in my hands, had been in my top drawer since I was twenty-two, and that was pure magic, and it was something worth staying alive for.

I picked up a book that had been recommended to me by a dear friend. *Traumata*, by Meera Atkinson, about sexual abuse and its aftermath. I found in her words the precise thing I had not been able to put into my own:

> I want to speak for those who grew up with family violence or dys-
> function and don't find a way out of the maze of substance addiction,

those who are diminished and die in trauma's long shadow, those who never find the words.

And I knew, then, something I couldn't have known without Meera, and Leslie, and Cheryl: that I might not be diminished and die in trauma's long shadow. That I might find the words, just like they had.

In 2019, I got a kitten. I knew that I needed something other than myself to stay alive for. Doesn't that sound selfish? It's hard to admit it. But it worked.

At the time, I was reading the novel *Eleanor Oliphant is Completely Fine*. In it, the protagonist adopts a cat immediately after her most serious suicide attempt. To honour all the destructive habits she is trying to beat, she calls the cat Glen, after the brand of vodka she drinks to excess every time she wants to die. The protagonist writes:

> Sometimes, after counselling sessions, I desperately wanted to buy vodka, lots of it, take it home and drink it down, but in the end I never did. I couldn't, for lots of reasons, one of which was that if I wasn't fit to, then who would feed Glen? She isn't able to take care of herself. She needs me. It isn't annoying, her need – it isn't a burden. It's a privilege. I'm responsible. I chose to put myself in a situation where I'm responsible.

I named my cat Glen, too, after Eleanor's. I no longer spend so much of my time actively thinking about suicide. During lockdown, I stopped drinking altogether. It only lasted two months, but it's something. It's a start. I learned that I really am strong enough to withstand my worst feelings without needing to numb them. Just like Dale, sobriety got me out of the boring prison my repetitive escapist behaviours had become.

I think fighting shame requires excruciating presence. That's not to say that sobriety is always the answer, or is right for everyone. But I do think there's a reason so many of us are drawn to it.

The false self, Dr Joseph Burgo tells us in his book *Shame*, is about escape. When shame is transmitted to us, we become convinced that our authentic self is somehow not good enough, somehow worthy of whatever shameless act we endured. So then our instinct is to escape that self. To hide from ourselves, to lie to ourselves, to erase the person we were when the first bad thing happened.

For some of us, that means becoming addicted to perfectionism. Becoming so busy and distracted we feel like we can outrun ourselves. Constantly seeking external markers of success to rewrite who we are.

But for some, that same impulse, the need to hide, gets expressed through drugs or alcohol or sex or eating or dieting or any other habit that gives us a way out. I think so many of the people in this book have used those addictions to quell shame. I certainly have.

I think understanding shame helps us understand the need to come back into ourselves and be present, either through sobriety or writing or just paying attention. I think that's a big part of getting better.

CHAPTER THIRTEEN

I think it's interesting that almost all of my interviews for this book about bodies also ended up being about relationships, about romance. But then again, of course they did. For women, the body is the vessel through which they give and receive love and intimacy – at least, something they are told is love and intimacy. The body is ground zero. They have to carry it through every relationship they build and every relationship they take apart, and it remembers every moment.

In Deborah Levy's memoir *The Cost of Living*, she perfectly captures the calculation women make when they decide to enter into certain kinds of heteronormative relationships. As her own marriage falls apart, Levy reflects on the home she has built for her family. The one she is leaving behind, taking apart in a weekend something that took twenty years to build.

She describes herself coming up for air after all these years and trying to will herself to swim back to the boat of her marriage. But she cannot do this.

Here's what she realizes in these moments, though. She has built a home for her family, yes. A home for her husband and children. But she has never found a way to build a home for herself, either within her body or outside of it.

Levy's disappointment is palpable. She writes that a lifetime of prioritizing the well-being of men and children leaves behind an 'unthanked, unloved, neglected, exhausted woman'. And so she poses the memoir's existential question: if women choose love, what does it cost them? And what price are they willing to pay?

I was drawn to the work because of the way it is able to express love, nostalgia and disappointment at the same time. When Levy reflects on her twenty years of marriage, she is heartbroken. The memories are fond and painful. They reverberate. But she is also clear-eyed and, ultimately, I think, hopeful. Hopeful that whether she decides to love again or not – she tells the reader that she has not made up her mind – she will do so knowing fully what price she is willing to pay, which sacrifices she is willing to make, and which she is not.

When I finally came up for air from the wreckage of my relationship, that's how I felt, too. Heartbroken, of course. Heartbroken then, heartbroken still. But happy in the knowledge that I had made a decision about the cost of love, and even though it was the most painful thing I have ever felt, I knew it was the right one. I had sacrificed too much, and all those sacrifices had come down to a fundamental belief that there was something shameful about me, something toxic. Walking away was an important part of realizing that belief was false.

But what I had given – time, energy, care, support – is still seen as something women can and should give away for free. The cost of intimacy is so much higher, simply because women's work has always been invisible, has been built into the idea of a relationship itself.

As she leaves, Levy's parting thought is:

> I will never stop grieving for my long-held wish for enduring love that does not reduce its major players to something less than they are. My shame had led me to accept a relationship that made me so much less than I am.

This, again, is what I love about this account. Levy's decision to leave her marriage is not about giving up on love. It is about believing it can be better.

.   .   .

It's almost summer when I meet Annabel. Her face pops up on my Zoom screen and her bedroom immediately catches my eye. It is beautiful. The duvet is bright white and there are several fluffy pillows and a thriving green houseplant is sitting next to her bed. Her room has a big window and the late May sun is pouring through it. I immediately think how together she is, how grown-up. She seems so composed. I have a moment of profound cognitive dissonance when she says, before anything else: Sorry about my bedroom, it's not exactly adult enough for a thirty-seven-year-old. And as with so many other moments of interpersonal connection I encountered while writing this book, it becomes clear that the way I see her and the way she sees herself do not overlap at all, not even close.

Annabel was twenty years old when she lost her mother. Everything felt heavy after that, and especially her body, her flesh. She had always been an ambitious girl, a vivacious teenager, but when her mother got sick all the fire in her seemed to dull.

Throughout the first years of her twenties, Annabel tried to focus on university and her friends and all the other things a girl of her age was supposed to focus on. But her focus always ended up coming back to the same place. She wanted to be smaller. To be less visible.

She started starving herself in earnest in her mid-twenties – something which, she acknowledges to me when we speak, is fairly unusual. A teenage-girl disease, people often think. But it struck Annabel just as hard at twenty-five as it had her school peers at fifteen. She developed more and more and more rules around food – things she could and couldn't eat, foods she could and couldn't touch, times of day when she could and could not think about food and her body. What she tells me now is something she did not recognize at twenty-five: that at the core of it, she was sad. She wanted, more than anything, to hurt herself, to enact her anger and hurt on something so it did not just sit inside her like lead.

Annabel's little sister had a very serious eating disorder, much more serious than her own, Annabel tells me. So she could constantly tell herself that her condition wasn't that bad, that it could always be worse.

Always hard-working and clever, Annabel worked in finance. She started out as a junior on a trading floor at one of the City of London's big banks, constantly weighing up risks and opportunities and serving clients as best she could. Wanting to please, aware that she was one of few women on her trading floor, Annabel was constantly trying to prove herself. She got to work early and stayed late. She pushed herself to do better and better on her work tasks, to become the best young trader in her firm. Every time she reached a goalpost, it shifted. Nothing was ever enough.

The high-stress environment of working in London finance fuelled her commitment to her eating disorder. Everything slotted together: constantly working gave her an excuse not to eat or think about food, and constantly being under pressure gave her an excuse for losing weight. As Annabel tells me this, I nod emphatically. I know this trick; I've used it a hundred times.

As a woman, it is easy to design a life around the principle of self-punishment. If you have that thing inside you, something telling you that you deserve it, then you can fashion an existence based on that feeling and very few people will question you or intervene. Because everyone else is taught that women deserve it, too.

After three exhausting years at the bank, Annabel was approached about a job at a new, innovative exchange in the City. Proud of herself, she accepted. The exchange was a smaller company than her bank, and the role was more senior, and she felt pleased. For a while, she felt less miserable; she even thought she might be able to get on top of her eating. But soon the new workplace revealed itself to be just as toxic as the last, and the pressure mounted, and the hours lengthened, and Annabel fell back into the same miserable feeling she had had the year before.

In the background to Annabel's inner turmoil, the world she knew was in tumult as well. In July, just after she had started her new job, the UK voted to leave the EU. Like so many on the left of politics, Annabel was shocked. It had seemed fairly certain that Remain would nudge out a victory, if only a small one, in the very worst-case scenario. What had been going on around her that she hadn't been paying attention to?

Just a few months later, Donald Trump was elected president in the US, and Annabel had that feeling again. She started thinking a lot about how the discontent that fed these upsets could ultimately be traced back to the financial crisis. The culmination of rampant capitalism, the idea that capital doesn't discriminate, that anyone can participate until the ship sinks and only the privately safety-netted survive.

Months and months of thinking this over left Annabel more discontent with her life than ever. She couldn't stop thinking about the fact that she worked for a corrupt banking system that had brought so many to their knees, brought them to a point of desperation that allowed them to be preyed upon by opportunistic stuntmen. She started thinking about how she could get out, but it felt almost impossible. She was in her mid-twenties and at the bottom of the ladder in what could be a stable career – how could she throw that away?

Without her noticing, Annabel's eating disorder got worse and worse. By the time she was thirty-three, she couldn't stop starving herself, couldn't stop purging, couldn't wrench back control of the thing she had originally taken up as a means of control itself.

She decided everything had to change. She had to blow up her life and start again. I know this feeling, I think as she talks. I did this, too, when I finally ran out of options, when my breakdown was too hard to come back from.

·   ·   ·

I feel so close to Annabel when I speak to her. It's because she is making me think of myself making a decision to change my life, reminding me how uncertain I was that it would work. For hours after we speak, I am lost in the memory.

I was twenty-five and sitting on the floor of the fourth living room I had shared with my partner over almost five years. I surveyed the damage of what seemed to me, in that moment, to be the graveyard of our life: half-packed boxes, half-empty bookshelves, a drawing I had commissioned for him for the first birthday of his that we'd shared, sitting on the floor, stripped from the wall where it had always been given pride of place. The co-parented cat who was looking longingly at me, puzzled, sad, wondering why I had torn his life apart.

It was as though the feeling in my chest might crush me from the inside out. I felt bereft. I *was* bereft. I had just lost the one thing I knew I was good at. But the price of being good at it had been too high, I know that now. But in that moment, I did not understand why I was doing what I was doing. I just knew that I no longer had a choice.

A close friend was waiting in her car outside. She was driving me and my ironing board to the room I was subletting until I found somewhere to live. I do not know why the ironing board was the only thing I took with me. Perhaps it had something to do with wanting to appear put together while shattering. Or maybe I'm just making that up now, as I write this. Memory is tricky.

As we drove, I was thinking about only one thing: If I am no longer a girlfriend, who will I be?

A few days later, I was on Tinder. I shouldn't have been, but I was, because I had fallen into the age-old trap of believing that pretending to be okay would make it so. The men I was speaking to kept asking me about my hobbies. What did I do for fun? I had no answer.

I told myself I would heal in that borrowed room, but I didn't. No one heals that quickly. So, months and months later, when I received a spreadsheet from my former partner cataloguing our life together, it destroyed me.

The spreadsheet had several rows listing all the things we had bought together. Cutlery, crockery, sofas, kettles, toasters, outdoor furniture for the balcony of that last apartment, the one that felt the most grown-up and held the most promise but also the one we knew from the beginning wouldn't last. The spreadsheet aimed to calculate what the relationship had cost us.

It had four columns. The first one was called 'item'. The second one 'full cost'. The third 'half cost'. And the fourth: 'depreciated half cost'.

The canonical thinker and writer Simone de Beauvoir spent most of her life in love with her male partner, Jean-Paul Sartre. But she refused, again and again, to enter into the kind of relationship he wanted. She refused to play the role of the wife, no matter how in love she was. On so many occasions throughout their lives, Sartre asked de Beauvoir to marry him, to move in with him, to start a family with him. But she couldn't. She didn't want to give up her writing life, her thinking life, to take on the role those things would demand of her.

As Levy writes: 'She knew it would cost her more than it would cost him. In the end she decided she couldn't afford it.'

In the end, she decided she couldn't afford it.

History is filled with women who are singled out for making this decision. When faced with the cost of intimacy, they turn away. Perhaps at this moment in history, there is a version of romantic love that does not cost us so much. Like Levy, I am hopeful.

When De Beauvoir was a child, she used to invent games to play with her sister based on Louisa May Alcott's *Little Women*. She would always play the role of Jo March – the second eldest in a set of four sisters living in Massachusetts in the 1860s, and the novel's heroine. Jo is the tomboy of the household. She is fiercely independent. She is also, importantly, a writer. Jo tells her reader she never wants to get married. She has already decided she cannot afford it.

De Beauvoir would always play Jo in her childhood games, because, she says, 'I was able to tell myself that I too was like her. I too would be superior and find my place.'

Susan Sontag also once told a journalist that she would never have become a writer had it not been for Jo March. Alcott had created a character that allowed women like de Beauvoir and Sontag to imagine the life they wanted – one that ended up being fulfilling without traditional romantic intimacy.

In *Little Women*, Alcott created a literary sensation for the ages. Since it was first published in 1868, it has never been out of print. I can't help but think that the thing drawing those readers to *Little Women* again and again was the same thing that drew de Beauvoir to it, that drew Sontag to it.

Alcott fashioned Jo March on herself. Alcott, like Jo, was a writer who saved her impoverished family by selling short stories to weekly magazines under a pseudonym.

Alcott, like Jo, was determined never to get married.

She kept her promise to herself: Alcott never married.

Alcott's own mother knew how high the cost of love could be. She both provided for and cared for her four girls as well as their father, Frank Alcott, who 'had ideas' and who considered himself a philosopher, but who never actually worked. He was distant and incompetent, and left the family poor and desperate and never felt the need to work or provide for them. Alcott never admired or liked her father, and I suspect she saw clearly just how much he drained and took advantage of her mother. Perhaps this is why her father was the one person who was left out of the family she created in *Little Women* – the four March girls live with their adored and adoring mother, but their father is away at war for the majority of the novel.

In one of the film adaptations of the novel, the director gives the March girls' mother, known as Marmee, a scene that is not in the book. One of the girls has twins and Marmee has to step in to be the midwife. As Joan Acocella writes in a piece in the *New Yorker*, 'How Little Women Got Big', in this scene we see in Marmee's face 'everything that Alcott hinted at but did not say about how her own mother was left to do everything'.

But while Alcott kept her promise to herself for life, she couldn't do the same for Jo. In Greta Gerwig's 2019 adaption of the novel, Jo's editor tells her that no one is interested in women's stories unless the girls 'end up dead or married'.

Unfortunately, Alcott found the same thing. She never intended to marry off Jo – she planned to give her the solitary writer's life she wanted so badly. But when Alcott published the first part of *Little Women*, she was flooded with letters from readers desperate to know who Jo ended up marrying, urging Alcott to give the girl a different kind of happy ending than the one she wanted.

Annabel quit her job at the exchange and decided to live off her savings while she tried to repair herself physically. She set herself a goal: to swim a mile in the River Thames.

She found a therapist and started trying to put on weight and get her profoundly disordered eating under control. She started exercising again. With every pound she put on, she felt her body get stronger. And with every ounce of strength, she felt her willingness to keep putting on weight grow bigger.

When she tells me this story, I am struck by a thought I have had over and over and over again while writing this book. We are always taught that success looks like big moments and breakthroughs, big achievements, stages, applause, promotions, weddings, books. But it isn't. The truth is that success is found in the tiniest increments, the smallest moments that build up to a new life.

At the height of her eating disorder, Annabel decided to leave the finance industry. She couldn't bear it any more; her mental health was crumbling by the day, and her body was disappearing, and she didn't have the strength to carry on. She had been functionally anorexic for all of the second half of her twenties. She needed to do something.

Quitting her job felt empowering and freeing, she tells me. As someone who also left a high-powered job in the middle of a breakdown, I know what she means. It's funny, because as Type A overachievers, opting out of something is the last thing either of us would ever have thought would bring us joy. But when our bodies forced us into it, it turns out that it did.

In the time after she left her job and before she started working again, Annabel started to think more clearly about the world around her. She thought about Brexit, and about Trump, and capitalism, and greed. She thought about her complicity in the industry she had been happy achieving in and making money in for so many years.

This structural thinking started to – slowly, but surely – change the way she felt about her body, too. Casting her mind outwards for the first time in years allowed her to start questioning what she really believed about body image.

I started reading all these books about the politics of space, she tells me. I just couldn't stop. I realized that my decision to minimize the space I take up, to hide myself away in a skeletal body, is a political act. And it's not one that I actually believe in at all.

She realized that part of her reckoning with the world and its broken systems would mean reckoning with the way those structures had played out on her own body.

All of a sudden, I desperately wanted to get on top of my eating disorder, she said.

For Annabel, the way to do this was to start thinking about her body as functional rather than aesthetic. She decided to start swimming again. She had always liked swimming, but she hadn't done it for years, and she hadn't had the energy for exercise since her early twenties – before she stopped eating. So she knew that in order to get back into the pool, she would need to start building muscle. To do that, she would need to eat.

Slowly, Annabel got used to the idea of eating regular-sized meals every day. It was painful and uncomfortable, but she kept doing it. Soon, she noticed she had started gaining weight and feeling stronger. She started doing small amounts of exercise to see what her body could handle, and she realized that for the first time in almost a decade, it could hold her up.

She started swimming every day and her arms and shoulders grew bigger with muscle and strength, and to her surprise, she was proud of this more often than she was ashamed.

The more she swam, the more she ate, and the more she ate, the more she swam. It's always the tiny habits that build up to a new body and a new life.

She got more serious about eating well after she had made the decision to swim a mile in the Thames, and she exercised more and more.

I wasn't going to be someone who had to get pulled out of the water halfway through the race by a surf lifesaver on a kayak, she says to me over Zoom. That is not going to be part of the story of my life.

I nod, because I know exactly how she feels.

Over the months that followed, Annabel says she went through something of a second puberty. My body completely changed at thirty-two, she says. I put on weight around my hips and arms and legs, and my face filled out.

It was so difficult to get used to, she tells me. I was getting strong, and there was muscle there, but there was also more cushioning than I had previously had on my jutting, hard-edged frame. I knew it was what I wanted, but there was still sometimes the voice in my head telling me I had failed at something important.

But she didn't give in to those voices. She kept training and she kept eating. She started a temp job at a domestic violence charity. She loved the team and the work they did so much that she kept temping until there was a full-time position available that she could apply for. It seemed to slot in with her new way of thinking about the world, and she loved how much the organization was committed to helping vulnerable women. She got the first full-time position that came up, and when I speak to her five years later, she is still working there.

Annabel successfully swam the Thames mile the next year, and she has swum it several times since then. She has also run two half-marathons and a number of smaller long-distance running competitions.

By the end of my relationship I had poured so much emotional energy into the project of creating and recreating my partner that I had no space left for me. He depended on me in those huge but invisible ways – for emotional support, for the steady hand to right the ship of his life when it threatened to sink, for the level head to solve every problem before it had even become one.

Because this labour is feminized, it is too often erased. It is not measured. It does not show up on the spreadsheet representing the last breath of a relationship. So women are taught, again and again, to think it does not have a cost. But it does.

Because intimacy is tied to caring, and so many heteronormative relationships end up with caring moving primarily in one direction, many women find themselves in the position of constantly giving intimacy but getting very little in return. It is the loneliest feeling in the world.

I think what we have always meant by a room of one's own is permission to refuse to hand out care and not be cared for in return. Permission to assert, to insist, that we are in fact better taken care of if we are alone, and if we reserve the energies for ourselves that we would have spent on our partner.

To be the subject of care, but not the object of it, is a particular kind of erasure. It leaves women feeling lonely and unseen. They become a vessel for something bigger. A carrier of the support he needs to thrive. The architect of the life he wants – every day building it a little higher, a little more stable, until he is exactly who he wants to be.

To me, this sense of erasure of self is at the heart of the manic pixie dream girl trope – the overplayed notion in films and television of a romance in which a man's life is changed by the sudden appearance of a magical, devoted woman, one who urges him to start living but who never gets a life of her own.

As I sit on the bus to and from work as I am contemplating leaving my relationship, I listen on repeat to Olivia Gatwood's poem, 'Manic Pixie Dream Girl':

> Let me build myself smaller than you.
> Let me apologize when I get caught acting bigger than you.
> Let me always wait for this.
> Let me work for this.

Let me work for this. In those words I felt a niggling truth about my life. That I had been working all this time, but I had been alone in it. That in the end, it would cost me more than it cost him.

I was so scared of being alone. But eventually, I realized that I was already alone, and facing that fact would bring me some degree of comfort.

As I was trying to convince myself to leave, I came across an article in the *New Statesman*, 'Maybe You Should Just Be Single', by the writer Laurie Penny. It was just after Valentine's Day 2017. In the first few paragraphs of the piece, Penny says: 'I think that it's usually better for women to be single. Particularly young women. Particularly straight young women. Not just "alright", not just "bearable" – actively better.'

This was a radical proposition to me. I had always assumed that being in a long-term relationship was a valid – perhaps primary – indicator of success. That if I could prove that I could find and keep love, I had achieved something. And that if I lost it, this would be a catastrophic failure.

What Penny made me realize was that my focus on the individual characteristics of my relationship and its discontents was misguided. The problem was structural, historical. I had always known the imbalance in my relationship was not my partner's fault – he is a good person, and a loving partner – but I could not talk myself out of the idea that the fault was mine. But the truth is that it was neither of us. It was everything we had been taught about love. The fact that

I ended up pouring all of my spare energy into encouraging my partner is not something he ever asked me to do. Not consciously, anyway.

It was just something I knew, without being told, was expected of me. It is part of the role constructed for me in a way that it is not for him. He never asked me to set aside my own needs for his. He never told me I couldn't see my friends as much. He never asked me to give up the things I love in order to make his life better. But that's what I did. And I couldn't even see that I was doing it, because I had made myself invisible.

bell hooks writes in *All About Love*: 'Men are especially inclined to see love as something they should receive without expending effort. More often than not they do not want to do the work that love demands.' The way that men have been raised and socialized means they come to see love as a prize, that finding a partner is where the work ends. For women, it is the beginning.

The work I am talking about is not solely, or even primarily, about domestic labour, although that is certainly a factor in many of these arrangements. In Rachel Cusk's essay collection *Coventry*, she dedicates a whole essay, 'Making Home', to this idea. She writes:

> Entering a house, I often feel that I am entering a woman's body, and that everything I do there will be felt more intimately by her than by anyone else… A home is powered by a woman's will and work.

But it wasn't for me. My partner did far more of the housework than I did. I left far too much of it to him.

Still, there were all the other ways I kept him afloat. The ways I watched his mental health patterns, told him to go for a run when he needed to, came home early when he was spiralling, told his friends to look after him when he wouldn't listen to me. Found the job he wanted to apply for. Told him he could do it. Read his application for him. Found him a hobby when he tired of the job. All the small and big ways I helped him hold it together. That is the work of caring.

And so often, we get only scraps of it in return. We have to do all that work for ourselves as well as for him, and when something has to give – in my experience, at least – it is us.

The long-term effect of playing this role is to become, in Deborah Levy's words in *The Cost of Living*, 'a minor character in one's own life'. We develop the sense of being valuable only for the role we play in another's life and success. An accessory.

In Gatwood's poem, the manic pixie dream girl reassures her male partner: *Don't worry – you are still the lead role. This is your love story, about the way I teach you to live.*

In the wake of her marriage breakdown, Levy is asked to make a list of the major and minor characters in one of her novels. This gets her thinking about the characters in her own life – a transition between fact and fiction that reflects Levy's own movement between her career as a novelist and her transition into memoir. Too often, when women look back on lives spent building love and its consequences, they find that they have moved into the background.

Watching a younger woman hold off a man's advances in the opening pages of the book, Levy reflects – with sadness, nostalgia and, I think, hope – on the woman's ability to stand steadfast in her alone-ness. 'It was not that easy to convey to him, a man much older than she was, that the world was her world, too,' she writes. 'It had not occurred to him that she might not consider herself to be the minor character and him the major character.' And then, crucially, the shift that I am learning to recognize between the individual and the systemic: 'She had unsettled a boundary, collapsed a social hierarchy, broken with the usual rules.'

I love watching this woman through Levy's eyes. Through the eyes of the woman who chose not to swim back to the boat. There is so much admiration there.

How many women become emotional carers because they believe in sunk costs, or because they believe it is their duty to believe in sunk costs?

In the end, my partner and I broke up on a Thursday. We got back together on a Tuesday. Then we broke up again. It was so hard to let each other go.

On that first Thursday, I was giving a presentation about intellectual property in my evening class at law school. All I could think about was the conversation I was going to have when I got home. My heart was already breaking; I could feel the pressure it was putting on my chest.

I had made the decision that I could no longer keep up my end of the bargain. I had decided that I had sacrificed too much in the creation of him, and as soon as that thought had crystallized in my mind, the relationship was over. Being a partner was the most important job I had ever had. I couldn't bear the thought of doing it badly. Not for another minute.

I had been so convinced, all my life, that the right thing to do was to stay. I don't know exactly where I got this from. I come from a long line of stoic women who have taken care of male partners, sometimes to their own detriment. Perhaps I learned it from them. But their feminist ideals were also the only reason I felt able to leave. The cognitive dissonance lived in me as strongly as it lived in them.

In those days leading up to the end of my relationship, though, I realized something. I had always believed that as a woman I had to do the right thing, which would invariably be to stay. The kind thing. The caring thing. But I cared too much about caring to do it half-heartedly, to disgrace its memory by being an unwilling participant, a minor character, in my own life.

So, I realized, the right thing is not always to stay. I could be more caring, and more kind, and more compassionate, both to my former partner and to the world, if I found a way to leave. I had to find a way to leave.

·　　·　　·

Annabel is thirty-seven when we speak, and she regularly competes in long swims and runs and is happy and fulfilled in her job. She has also taken the leap of adding another bucket list item to her list of recent achievements: she has completed an MA in English litera-ture, something she has always wanted to do but never given herself permission for.

But one thing I'm still working on, she says, is how to see my new body sexually again. It is so ingrained in my mind that the only kind of body that will ever be desired is my smallest, most diminished one. I'm still trying to convince myself that I can engage with myself sexually and engage with my desire now that I am bigger.

I ask her to tell me more about this.

It just feels like the last hurdle, you know, she says.

And I do. I do know.

So I kind of decided to cut myself off from engaging in sex or dating for years and years, while I was trying to get better, she adds.

Me too, I say.

And it really helped, she says. I honestly don't think I would have had the emotional energy to date or have a relationship during my recovery. I hate how much pressure we are under as women to find relationships in order to be fulfilled.

I nod my head so hard I worry it might fall off.

Annabel continues: People are always asking me if I'm dating, when I'll start dating again, *you're not getting any younger*, they say. And I know that, but who are they to presume that romance is a priority for me? It just isn't.

I nod even more.

So I decided that maybe it's also a political act to remove yourself from that space, she says.

YES, I shout at the Zoom screen.

So it's been years since I was intimate with anyone, she tells me, but I've realized recently that I'm finally becoming comfortable with my own sexuality and my body again.

That's great, I say, and I remember that I had meant to ask her what her MA research was on.

It's on women poets and the politics of solitude, she says. I'm actually starting a PhD on it in September.

.　　.　　.

After my partner moved out, the apartment haunted me. Our cat was confused. Every night I got home from work exhausted, crushed, hungover, spent, and I said to him: It's just you and me now. I wasn't sure if I was explaining this to him or reinforcing it in my own mind, knowing how much I desperately wanted to swim back to the boat.

The pain of it was almost unbearable. It was unlike anything I had ever felt. The trauma of separation tore at me. I missed him. I wanted him to come home. Sometimes I still do. After all my intellectualizing of my role in the world, after all my rethinking about structures and agency and love, I regress to my most fundamental desire: I just want to fix it.

I stopped sleeping. I lay awake all night watching the *Sex and the City* movie and thinking about how I would never fall in love again. I drank red wine and I swallowed temazepam, but still I could not sleep.

The truth was I had been alone for a long time. The truth was I had been wholly invested in something he had never quite committed to, not really. The truth was I had lost myself in him.

The truth was I wanted to put my needs before anyone else's, for the first time in my life.

I struggled so much with the ethics of this. Who would I be if I forfeited that responsibility? I spoke to my therapist, my sister, my friends. I tried to measure our faults in the relationship. Could I justify it? Could I give a list of transgressions as evidence of my moral right to leave? Would it hold up under scrutiny?

In the end it didn't matter. I wanted a different life for myself. I couldn't think my way out of that.

Levy writes that 'chaos is supposed to be what we most fear, but I have come to believe it might be what we most want.' It might be, she says, the thing that brings us closer to how we want to be in the world.

Cheryl Strayed writes in her piece 'The Truth that Lives There', 'Go, because you want to. Because wanting to leave is enough.' What a radical proposition that was – at least to me. *Wanting to leave is enough.*

What I discovered after leaving my relationship was that caring energy is finite. Once I had stopped caring for him, I became able to care for myself for the first time. Sometimes I am still ashamed of this, but mostly I am proud of it.

I started writing more. I started writing all the time. I wrote my first book. Then I wrote this one – my second.

Laurie Penny writes in the *New Statesman* about two versions of herself – the one she can be while partnered and the one she can be while she is alone. 'That self,' she writes, 'the self that was dedicated to writing, travelling and doing politics, that had many outside interests and more intense friendships, was not something men seemed to value or desire.'

Could that be true? Had I suppressed the part of me that was dedicated to writing in order to be a better partner, to live up to my own standard of womanly commitment? Was that part of my false self, the self that needed to change in order to be loved? I can't be sure, even now. But something had definitely changed.

Could the caring that is poured into writing be a kind of caring for the self – the kind I did not discover until I stopped swimming back to the boat?

Is it a coincidence that Jo March and Susan Sontag and Simone de Beauvoir felt they had to make a choice between love – of a certain kind – and writing?

Another thing I discovered is that an arrangement where intimacy is given but not received in return leads to a particular kind of isolation. So many men who are the subjects of this intimacy believe they deserve to have it exclusively. The structural expectation is that women reserve their intimate selves for men, even though their own intimate selves are starving. Women become less and less able to seek that same intimacy from friends and family because of that same sense of duty.

When I left my relationship, I leaned on my friends wholly. I collapsed onto them. Collectively and individually, they bore the weight of my grief. I have never felt so cared for. Years on from those weeks and months, my caring relationship with them is just as strong.

Almost two years to the day after my relationship ended for the final time, I was packing my things into boxes in a small, almost windowless flat in Finsbury Park in North London. I had lived here since I had walked away from my old life in Sydney. It's something I had always wanted to do, and here I was.

The flat was airless and stuffy and small, but I loved it. It was the first time I had ever truly lived on my own, and it is all I had ever wanted. When I took the flat I was new to London and did not have a real job – only a book contract and a promise to pay the rent. It was all I could afford.

But on this day, in August 2019, I had just been offered and had accepted a well-paid job as a journalist to support my writing and to pay the rent. So I was moving into a bigger flat – with windows and a spare room. A room to write.

It was among the proudest moments of my life, this moving day. It felt like an almost endless series of tiny, heart-wrenching steps away from something had led me, finally, to something else. Something that glimmered with hope. Perhaps this is why I found so much hope in the pages of Levy's memoir.

I listened to Levy's book on audio as I packed up my stuffy flat. Everything she said about the cost of love shattered and rebuilt me. It was everything I had been thinking for these last years, put into words in a way I could never have fathomed, on a day that seemed so symbolic.

Perhaps chaos is the thing that brings us nearer to who we want to be in the world. It certainly was for me.

But here is the most important thing. After everything she has experienced, Levy writes that 'to separate from love is to live a risk-free life… What's the point of that sort of life?'

She still believes. So do I.

Walking away from a particular kind of love does not mean giving up on it. Quite the opposite. It is learning what we can afford to pay for it and what we can't. And that means that when we approach it again, it will be with conviction.

I am not giving up on love. I am demanding a better version of it. A version of myself in love that I can live with.

As I was packing up my things that day, I listened to Levy describe her own process of moving out of her family home and into a new, post-marriage flat. She describes the space as both eerie and comforting. It was new and full of possibility. She describes writing books on the balcony and renaming the creepily lit hallways as the 'corridors of love'. She was happy even though she was heartbroken, I can tell. I have been there.

I began to sentimentalize the fact that I was moving house just as Levy – or the version of her narrating her audiobook in that moment – was moving house. To romanticize everything is an instinct I cannot tame.

But as she described the building on the top of a hill in North London, with art deco interiors and a 1930s council flat exterior, I began to think about how much it really did sound like the building I was moving into later that day.

The next morning, I was chatting in the lift to a fellow resident. I was elated and full of purpose, walking to the plant shop in Crouch End again and again to show my new flat how committed I was to it.

I was holding Levy's memoir in my hands as I emptied out my handbag, searching for my keys.

Ah, my lift-mate said. Did you know she lives in this building?

REACTIONS IN THE AFTERMATH

a list in ~~three~~ four parts

4

Three or more years, ten years, a lifetime after:

· Vulnerability, by which I mean strength

ACKNOWLEDGEMENTS

This book belongs to so many people. First and foremost, to all the people I interviewed for this book: thank you for sharing your stories with me. I will never forget the time we spent together. Your generosity and openness in our conversations and your willingness to work with me to get these stories right is absolutely astounding, and I will always be indebted to you for that.

To my agent, Emma Paterson, who has been there for me every step of the way and without whose help I would be totally, utterly lost. Thank you, Emma, for all you have done for me and for making sure this book made it out into the world. I owe you so much.

To Susie, Alex and the whole team at The Indigo Press – thank you for all of your incredible guidance throughout this process and for being so supportive and understanding. Thank you for commissioning this book and believing in it when I did not, and thank you for continuing to offer me that support every step of the way.

Thank you so much to Gillian, who was just the most brilliant editor and did just a wonderful job of bringing this book to life. Gillian's excellent literary guidance as well as fierce emotional support was a lifeline for me this past year.

Thank you to Ellah Wakatama Allfrey, who made this book possible and whose belief in me has been unfailing and so magical. Without you, Ellah, none of this would have happened. I will never be able to thank you enough for believing me and giving me the chance of a lifetime.

Thank you to Kelly, Is and to everyone at Allen & Unwin for your editorial support and guidance and your belief in me. I am so lucky to be able to work with you, and I am so grateful to you. Our book tour at the beginning of 2020 and all of your support in publicizing *I Choose Elena* was one of the things that made me feel as though this book was possible.

To Sarah T and Alex and everyone who helped with the production of this book, thank you from the bottom of my heart. Thank you for your incredible skill and diligence as well as your understanding, compassion and sensitivity.

Thank you to my friends and family, who put up with all the tears I cried while trying to get this book right. Thank you to everyone who supported me through this process and was willing to be there to help with my writing woes in the middle of a global pandemic. You are all shining lights. Thank you.

BIBLIOGRAPHY

Alexander, Michelle, *The New Jim Crow: Mass Incarceration in the Age of Colorblindness* (The New Press, 2010).

Atkinson, Meera, *Traumata* (University of Queensland Press, 2018), pp. 22, 60.

Barrett, Lisa Feldman, *How Emotions Are Made: The Secret Life of the Brain* (Picador, 2017).

Best, Clare, *The Missing List* (Linen Press, 2018), location 595 (Kindle edition).

Boon, Suzette, *Coping with Trauma-Related Dissociation: Skills Training for Patients and Therapists* (W.W. Norton & Company, 2011).

Borysenko, Joan, *Minding the Body, Mending the Mind* (Hay House, 2005).

Boyer, Anne, *The Undying* (Allen Lane, 2019), p. 67.

Bradshaw, John, *Healing the Shame That Binds You* (Health Communications Inc EB, 2010), p. 738.

Brown, Brené, *I Thought It Was Just Me: Women Reclaiming Power and Courage in a Culture of Shame* (Gotham Books, 2007).

Brown, Brené, *Men, Women and Worthiness: The Experience of Shame and the Power of Being Enough* (Health Communications Inc, 2005; Sounds True, 2012).

Burgo, Joseph, *Why Do I Do That? Psychological Defense Mechanisms and the Hidden Ways They Shape Our Lives* (New Rise Press, 2012).

Burgo, Joseph, *Shame: Free Yourself, Find Joy, and Build True Self-Esteem* (St Martin's Press, 2018).

Doidge, Norman, *The Brain's Way of Healing: Stories of Remarkable Recoveries and Discoveries* (Penguin, 2015).

Eddo-Lodge, Reni, *Why I'm No Longer Talking to White People About Race* (Bloomsbury Circus, 2017).

Engel, Beverly, *It Wasn't Your Fault: Freeing Yourself from the Shame of Childhood Abuse with the Power of Self-Compassion* (New Harbinger Publications, 2015).

Engeln, Renee, *Beauty Sick: How the Cultural Obsession with Appearance Hurts Girls and Women* (HarperAudio, 2017).

Epstein, Mark, *The Trauma of Everyday Life* (Penguin, 2013).

Evaristo, Bernardine, *Girl, Woman, Other* (Penguin, 2020), p. 338.

Farrow, Ronan, *Catch and Kill: Lies, Spies, and a Conspiracy to Protect Predators* (Little, Brown and Company, 2019).

Fisher, Janina, *Healing the Fragmented Selves of Trauma Survivors: Overcoming Internal Self-Alienation* (Routledge, 2017).

Gleeson, Sinead, *Constellations* (Picador, 2019), pp. 7, 50.

Gordon, James, *The Transformation: Discovering Wholeness and Healing After Trauma* (HarperOne, 2019).

Grace, Annie, *This Naked Mind: Control Alcohol, Find Freedom, Discover Happiness & Change Your Life* (HarperCollins, 2018).

Grayling, A.C., *Wittgenstein: A Very Short Introduction* (Oxford University Press, 2001).

Grisel, Judith, *Never Enough: The Neuroscience and Experience of Addiction* (Doubleday, 2019).

Heller, Lawrence, *Healing Developmental Trauma: How Early Trauma Affects Self-Regulation, Self-Image, and the Capacity for Relationship* (North Atlantic Books, 2012).

Herman, Judith, *Trauma and Recovery: The Aftermath of Violence – From Domestic Abuse to Political Terror* (Basic Books, 2015).

hooks, bell, *All About Love* (WmMorrowPB, 2015), p. 147.

Honeyman, Gail, *Eleanor Oliphant Is Completely Fine* (HarperCollins, 2017), p. 337

Hopper, Briallen, *Hard to Love: Essays and Confessions* (Bloomsbury, 2019), pp. 5, 9, 10, 22.

Jacquet, Jennifer, *Is Shame Necessary? New Uses for an Old Tool* (Pantheon, 2015).

Jamison, Leslie, *The Empathy Exams: Essays* (Granta Books, 2015), pp. 11, 204.

Jamison, Leslie, *The Recovering: Intoxication and Its Aftermath* (Little, Brown and Company, 2018).

Jamison, Leslie, *Make It Scream, Make It Burn: Essays* (Little, Brown and Company, 2019).

Kantor, Jodi, *She Said: Breaking the Sexual Harassment Story That Helped Ignite a Movement* (Penguin, 2019).

Karen, Robert, 'Shame', in *The Atlantic Monthly*, February 1992, pp. 40–70.

Kendall, Mikki, *Hood Feminism: Notes from the Women That a Movement Forgot* (Viking, 2020).

Khákpour, Porochista, *Sick: A Memoir* (Canongate Books, 2018).

Krasnostein, Sarah, *The Trauma Cleaner: One Woman's Extraordinary Life in Death, Decay and Disaster* (Text Publishing, 2018).

Laing, Olivia, *The Lonely City* (Canongate Books, 2016), pp. 3, 279.

Lee, Bri, *Eggshell Skull* (Allen & Unwin, 2018).

Levine, Peter, *Sexual Healing: Transforming the Sacred Wound* (Sounds True, 2003).

Levine, Peter, *In an Unspoken Voice: How the Body Releases Trauma and Restores Goodness* (North Atlantic Books, 2010).

Levine, Peter, *Trauma and Memory: Brain and Body in a Search for the Living Past* (North Atlantic Books, 2015).

Levine, Peter, *Waking the Tiger: Healing Trauma* (Tantor Media, 2016).

Levy, Deborah, *The Cost of Living* (Penguin, 2019), pp. 3, 7, 8, 94, 98.

Lorde, Audre, *Sister Outsider: Essays and Speeches* (Crossing Press, 1984).

Lorde, Audre, *Conversations With Audre Lorde* (University Press of Mississippi, 2004).

Lorde, Audre, *Your Silence Will Not Protect You* (Silver Press, 2017).

Lorde, Audre, *The Master's Tools Will Never Dismantle the Master's House* (Penguin Classics, 2018).

Machado, Carmen Maria, *In the Dream House: A Memoir* (Graywolf Press, 2019).

Maté, Gabor, *In the Realm of Hungry Ghosts: Close Encounters with Addiction* (Knopf Canada, 2007).

Maté, Gabor, *Close Encounters with Addiction* (Central Recovery Press, 2016).

Maté, Gabor, *The Return to Ourselves: Trauma, Healing, and the Myth of Normal* (Sounds True, 2018).

Maté, Gabor, *When the Body Says No: The Cost of Hidden Stress* (Vermilion, 2019).

Miller, Chanel, *Know My Name: A Memoir* (Viking, 2019).

Mills, Sam, *Chauvo-Feminism: On Sex, Power and #MeToo* (The Indigo Press, 2021), p. 25.

Nelson, Maggie, *The Argonauts* (Melville House UK, 2016), pp. 9, 140.

Odell, Jenny, *How to Do Nothing: Resisting the Attention Economy* (Melville House, 2019).

Offill, Jenny, *Dept. of Speculation* (Granta, 2015), pp. 8, 66.

Ogden, Pat, Kekuni Minto and Clare Pain, *Trauma and the Body: A Sensorimotor Approach to Psychotherapy* (W.W. Norton, 2006).

Orbach, Susie, *Fat Is A Feminist Issue* (Arrow, 2006).

Orbach, Susie, *Bodies* (St Martin's Press, 2009), p. 61.

Peletz, Michael G., *Gender Pluralism: Southeast Asia Since Early Modern Times* (Routledge, 2009), p. 22.

Price, Rosie, *What Red Was* (Vintage Digital, 2019).

Rich, Adrienne, *Adrienne Rich's Poetry and Prose* (W.W. Norton, 1993).

Rich, Adrienne, *On Lies, Secrets, and Silence: Selected Prose 1966–1978* (W.W. Norton, 1995), pp. 187, 189, 190, 191.

Ronson, Jon, *So You've Been Publicly Shamed* (Riverhead Books, 2015).

Rooney, Sally, *Conversations with Friends* (Faber & Faber, 2017), pp. 159, 162, 263.

Rothschild, Babette, *The Body Remembers: The Psychophysiology of Trauma and Trauma Treatment* (W.W. Norton, 2000).

Saad, Layla F, *Me and White Supremacy: Combat Racism, Change the World, and Become a Good Ancestor* (Sourcebooks, 2020).

Scarry, Elaine, *The Body in Pain* (Oxford University Press, 1987), p. 7.

Storr, Will, *Selfie: How the West Became Self-Obsessed* (Picador, 2017).

Storr, Will, *The Science of Storytelling* (William Collins, 2019).

Strayed, Cheryl, *Tiny Beautiful Things* (Atlantic Books, 2013).

Taddeo, Lisa, *Three Women* (Simon & Schuster, 2019).

Tolentino, Jia, *Trick Mirror: Reflections on Self-Delusion* (Random House, 2019), pp. 13, 15.

Twist, Jos, Ben Vincent, Meg-John Barker and Kat Gupta (eds), *Non-Binary Lives – An Anthology of Intersecting Identities* (Jessica Kingsley Publishers, 2020).

Vaid-Menon, Alok, *Beyond the Gender Binary* (Penguin Workshop, 2020), p. 20.

van der Kolk, Bessel, *The Body Keeps the Score: Mind, Brain and Body in the Transformation of Trauma* (Penguin Random House, 2015).

Walker, Pete, *Complex PTSD: From Surviving to Thriving* (Azure Coyote Publishing, 2013).

Windust, Jamie, *In Their Shoes: Navigating Non-Binary Life* (Jessica Kingsley Publishers, 2020).

Winnicott, Donald, *Maturational Processes and the Facilitating Environment* (Routledge, 1990), p. 187.

Wolynn, Mark, *It Didn't Start with You: How Inherited Family Trauma Shapes Who We Are and How to End the Cycle* (Viking, 2016).

Transforming a manuscript into the book
you hold in your hands is a group project.

Lucia would like to thank everyone who helped
to publish *My Body Keeps Your Secrets*.

THE INDIGO PRESS TEAM

Susie Nicklin
Alex Spears
Phoebe Barker
Honor Scott

JACKET DESIGN

Laura Thomas
Andy Soameson

FOREIGN RIGHTS

The Marsh Agency

PUBLICITY

Jordan Taylor-Jones

EDITORIAL PRODUCTION

Gillian Stern
Tetragon
Sarah Terry
Alex Middleton